Keep your
Senses Sharp

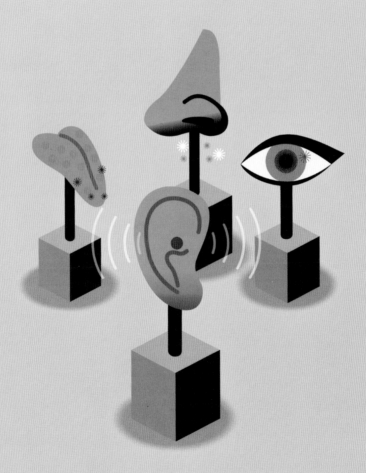

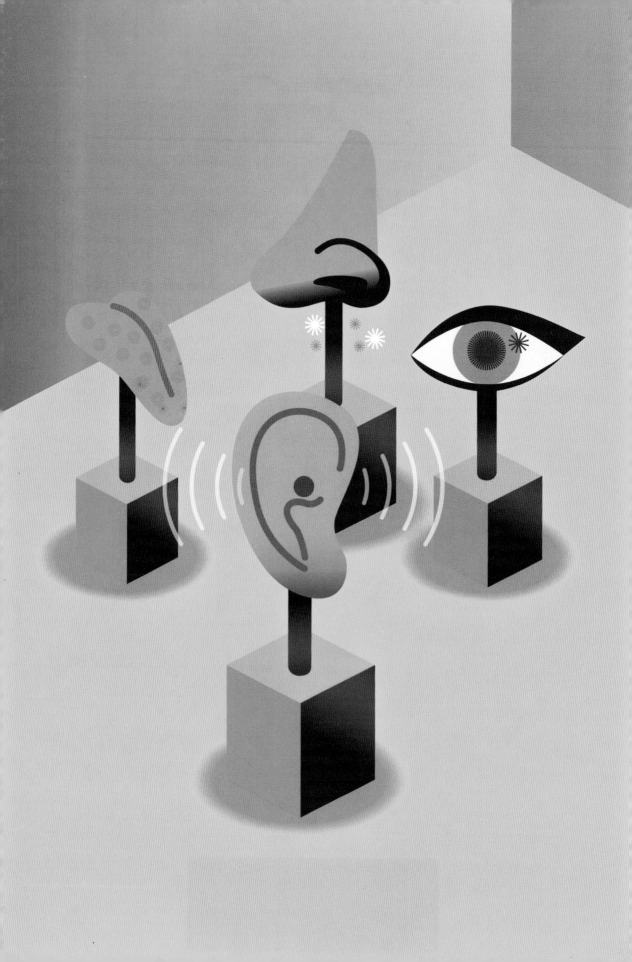

READER'S DIGEST **HEALTH SOLUTIONS**

Keep your Senses Sharp

How to preserve your eyesight, hearing, taste and smell and keep them working well

Published by Reader's Digest Association Ltd
London • New York • Sydney • Montreal

contents

expert consultants

Professor Ian Grierson PhD FRC Path
Professor of Ophthalmology
Unit of Ophthalmology and St Paul's Eye Unit
University of Liverpool

Matthew Yung MS PhD FRCS DLO
Consultant Otologist
The Ipswich Hospital NHS Trust

Dr Lucy Donaldson BDS BSc PhD
Senior Lecturer in Physiology and Pharmacology
School of Medical Sciences
University of Bristol

Professor Tim Jacob BSc PhD
Professor of Cell Physiology
School of Biosciences
Cardiff University

Writer
Sheena Meredith MB BS

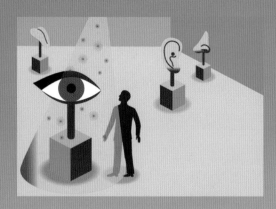

Sight

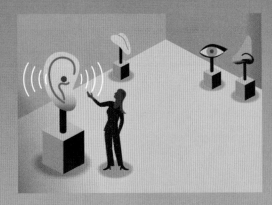

Hearing

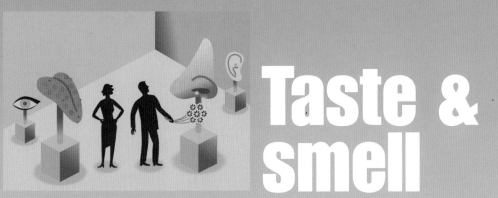

Taste & smell

about this book

Here is a book that can help you to live not just a healthy life but also one that is packed with enjoyment. *Keep your Senses Sharp* is about protecting and correcting senses that are as pleasurable as they are essential for our safety and everyday existence.

Many people accept without question that the senses get duller with age. But this is not inevitable. The book explains how to forestall the effects of ageing and also how to compensate for any impairment; thanks to new medical techniques and 21st-century technology, there is almost always something that can be done.

The book also outlines dozens of self-help measures that can make a real difference and explains in simple terms how the senses function, what can go wrong with them, tell-tale symptoms of damaging disorders, and when and where to seek help. You'll discover which lifestyle and environmental influences can damage eyesight, hearing, taste and smell, and how to avoid and combat them.

Most significantly, in each of the three sections – Sight, Hearing, Taste & smell – the book helps you to develop a personal action plan for preserving these senses for life.

your smart sense plan

Throughout, you'll see references to the *Smart Sense Plan* – a general programme for all your senses. It's made up of four elements – Protect, Assess, Correct and Enjoy (PACE) – this strategy is not just a progressive plan but also an indication of everything you can do to preserve and enhance your senses all the time. At the end of each section you'll find questions and page references to highlight specific pieces of advice.

Protect You'll discover the lifestyle choices that can help you to maintain and sharpen your senses, guard against future problems and deal with any that have already occurred. Some advice may sound familiar – cut back on animal fats, enjoy colourful fruits and vegetables, give up smoking. Like the rest of your body, your senses benefit from a healthy lifestyle. You'll learn how other aspects of the way we live – from computers to MP3 players – can adversely affect the senses, why eyes need darkness and ears need silence, and how you can sharpen your senses of taste and smell by simply indulging them.

Assess You need to know your starting point. How good is your sight? How well can you hear, or taste, or smell? What are you already doing to compensate – and is it effective? It's vital to know how well your senses are functioning and to be alert to any changes. You need to understand how each sense works, what might go wrong or get worse, and how likely that is, so that you can take action to prevent or treat any problems. You'll learn about risk factors and how some personal characteristics can make you more (or less) susceptible to certain disorders. Checklists and practical home experiments will help you to identify problems and decide whether you need to consult a GP or other specialist. And this is all advice that is valid at any time. Your *Smart Sense Plan* is a life-long strategy, with plenty of opportunities to assess and re-assess along the way.

Correct So often, disorders affecting the senses have a treatable cause, or there are effective ways to minimise their impact and continue to enjoy your work, hobbies, relationships to the full and to maintain your independence. *Keep your Senses Sharp* explains what you can do to correct a range of disorders that affect the senses and how to compensate for any loss or deterioration as you get older. Each section outlines what professional medical help is available and helps you to evaluate the treatments, strategies, gadgets and technical assistance that specialists may recommend.

Enjoy Our senses afford us endless delight – something we tend to overlook in the bustle of everyday life. To appreciate them to the full, we need to stop and look at whatever gives us pleasure, to listen to sounds that thrill us, to enjoy a beautiful fragrance or aroma, and to savour tastes that please our palate. Using them consciously also heightens our awareness. We notice more, we listen more discerningly, we refine our senses of taste and smell – which further enhances the enjoyment they bring. That pleasure should be a strong incentive to take care of our senses, protect and preserve them – for life.

Nobody should take their senses for granted. There is every reason to want to keep them working well. Devising a *Smart Sense Plan* that is right for you brings immediate benefits and will help you to continue to enjoy life to the full. The wealth of information and guidance in *Keep your Senses Sharp* could help you to preserve your independence and your zest for life well into old age.

introduction

Our senses are what connect us with the world. Without them, we would have no idea what's going on around us, no ability to navigate our environment, manage our affairs or enjoy life's pleasures, and no contact with other people.

Yet most of us take them for granted – most of the time. Think of the sensory coordination required to perform a simple action, such as answering a telephone. You need to hear it ringing, identify the nature and direction of the sound, locate the telephone by sight, walk over to it and touch and pick up the receiver. The action is largely unconscious – your mind is probably focused on who is calling or on the activity from which you were interrupted when the phone rang.

A SENSE OF JOY

Our senses are much more than mere mechanical aids. From the glories of orchestral music to the sudden appearance of the sun from behind a cloud, or the taste of chocolate to the smell of freshly-baked bread, our senses help us to enjoy life.

They can also evoke powerful emotions – the sight of a road accident or a newborn baby, the sound of a loved one's voice from afar, the smell of new-mown grass or of rotting food. Positive or negative, they mediate our experience of the world, sometimes beyond conscious awareness. Where does that sense of déjà vu come from? Why do you walk into your child's primary school and become instantly transported back to your own school days? How do those tunes arise and suddenly play in our heads?

SENSING TROUBLE

Our senses can thrill us, scare us, attract us or transport us back in time or place. Perhaps because of these magical qualities, we forget that they're physical functions which, like the rest of our bodies, require care and attention to work at their best. You may make an effort to keep your weight down, to eat healthily, or to avoid pollution, pesticides and additives, or to take regular exercise – but the chances are, you've never given a lot of thought to the health of your eyes and ears, never mind your nose and tongue.

We seldom take action until something goes wrong. It's only when you have to ask someone else to read the restaurant menu for you that you think, maybe, it's time for an eye test. Or loved ones whom you accuse of mumbling suggest that your hearing may be the problem – and that you turn up the TV volume far too loud. Food may not taste as good as it once did; roses may not smell as sweet. Too often we fail to notice the gradual changes that creep up on us as we reach middle age – and some people are simply not prepared to admit it, to themselves or anyone else.

THE RISKS OF NEGLECTING OUR SENSES

It is equally worrying that many people also accept such experiences as inevitable and a normal part of ageing. As this book shows, you don't have to. There are now many medical solutions to failing senses and, with something like sight, potentially blinding conditions – such as glaucoma – can be cured, if caught early enough.

Doing nothing can have serious consequences – needless loss of vision, for example, or the isolation and misery than comes from not being able to communicate with the people dearest to us. Having impaired senses can be dangerous too – putting us at greater risk of road accidents, or trips and falls, or the kitchen catching fire because we couldn't smell a smouldering meal or hear a smoke alarm.

Yet simple changes – from a new prescription for glasses to better lighting on the stairs – can often make a vast difference in improving both our safety and our quality of life.

The three sections of this book – Sight, Hearing, Taste & smell – provide all the information, tools and advice you need to take action early, avoid unforeseen consequences, and keep your senses in good working order. The wealth of information and guidance in *Keep your Senses Sharp* will help you to safeguard your senses, spot and get treatment for sense-threatening ailments, and preserve your independence and enjoyment of life into old age.

A PERSONAL PLAN

Most importantly, the book will also help you to develop your own *Smart Sense Plan* to maintain and preserve your senses of sight, hearing, taste and smell, and keep them in peak condition. A simple acronym – PACE – sums up the four key elements of the plan: Protect, Assess, Correct and Enjoy.

The plan includes tips and self-help strategies touching on diet and general lifestyle that will help you to safeguard and even enhance your senses, as well as warnings about the harmful influence of environmental factors, such as pervasive noise.

It outlines ways you can assess your own senses and the wide range of medical tests that GPs and specialists will carry out to pinpoint any problems. It takes you step-by-step through corrective techniques and reveals cutting-edge research that is paving the way for future cures. It also includes some fascinating case histories of people who, with the help of medical science or technology, have triumphed against the odds.

Enjoying your senses is, of course, the guiding principle of the book and the underlying purpose of the *Smart Sense Plan*. Our senses are the most pleasurable tools for living that we have, and actively using and appreciating them can play a vital role in preserving them.

But they are not a constant – they evolve and change over the years, so it's important to monitor your plan and its success as you go along. There will always be aspects that can be improved upon or modified.

USE OR LOSE ...

The importance of consciously using and monitoring our senses was highlighted by Professor Charles Spence of the Department of Experimental Psychology at the University of Oxford, in his 2002 ICI Report on the 'Secrets of the Senses'. In it, he warned that we are living in an age when our senses are simultaneously bombarded and deprived, which is potentially damaging to our health and well-being.

We have moved, he explains, from the largely outdoor, physical lifestyle of our ancestors to one in which we spend 90 per cent of our time indoors, often watching television or using computers. We overdose on information presented to our visual senses, but neglect the emotional senses of touch and smell – and we do so at our peril. The imbalance is affecting people's capacity for pleasure, love, success and a healthy life.

As a result, he says, we are also losing our senses of taste and smell more quickly, leading to possibly serious health and dietary problems in old age. We don't get enough touch stimulation to our skin and, according to Professor Spence, touch is not only essential for emotional well-being, but also for sensory, cognitive, neurological and physical development. Modern living has created a 'touch hungry' generation.

INDULGE YOURSELF

The solution? Sensory self-indulgence, says Professor Spence. We need to understand that our senses are intended to interact and work in harmony – and we need to incorporate that into our everyday experiences. We need more background smells, mood-enhancing music and tactile surfaces. We need to touch each other more. According to Professor Spence, indulgence is not hedonistic excess, but a deep biological need that fuels the development of our senses and aids health and happiness in later life.

Boosting all our senses will make us more productive, successful and able to enjoy moe fulfilling relationships, he says. What better justification could you want?

COMPENSATORY SENSES

If you need further evidence that the senses form a coordinated system, think about what happens to people who lose one of them. Helen Keller, the American author who was deaf and blind from babyhood, described how others were often surprised that she enjoyed the natural world. Yet she felt it was they who were really blind, for when sight is taken away the remaining senses truly come alive, in a manner incomprehensible to a sighted person. 'For they have no idea how fair the flower is to the touch, nor do they appreciate its fragrance, which is the soul of the flower.'

It's a widely held belief that when one major sense fails, others become super-sensitive to compensate. For example, deaf people are better able to detect vibration and movement, blind musicians have better pitch discrimination than sighted ones – and indeed it is believed that similar phenomena occur in animals.

But is it true? Some scientists suggest that it is not so much heightened sensitivity but more a case of heightened awareness and experience. When people have to rely on their other senses, they learn to use those senses more effectively, and perhaps their perception (how sensory information is interpreted in the brain) is altered, rather than their sensation.

This explanation matters because, if it's even partly down to attention and practice, that implies that anyone can boost their sensory experiences and expertise – which is just what Professor Spence recommends.

A WEALTH OF SENSES

Here's something else intriguing. We are traditionally taught that we have five senses: vision, hearing, touch, taste and smell, a classification believed to have been devised by Aristotle.

In fact there are more, though because there is no uniform definition of what constitutes a 'sense', different scientists discuss different numbers of senses.

Some scientists separate vision into two or even three senses, on the basis that colour, brightness and perhaps depth are all sensed by different mechanisms.

Similarly, both taste and smell can be subdivided according to the different receptors used to detect different smells or tastes. As well as receptors in taste buds on our tongue, we have other chemical sensors in our mouth and throat that contribute to flavour by detecting heat and cool sensations from food, as well as the 'wow' factor of spices like chilli.

In the same way, we have two types of touch sensation relying on pressure sensors in the skin, one for light touch and one for deep pressure. And we have sense receptors in our skin for temperature, itch and pain – our pain sense can distinguish between mechanical, heat and chemical threats. As these rely on different receptors, some experts argue that they should be considered as separate senses.

INSIDE-OUTSIDE

In addition, while our basic five senses communicate information about the environment outside the body, most scientists include at least two other senses that rely on communications from within the body and are responsible for balance and awareness of body position. Others would say that sensations such as hunger and thirst were 'senses', too.

MAKING SENSE OF THE WORLD

Whatever they are, this wealth of senses filters our experiences of the world. The sense itself may prompt an instant reflex reaction, as when we withdraw our hand quickly from a flame, even before our brain determines the potential for a burn. But usually incoming sensory stimulation is then processed by the brain to create our perceptions – along with memory and understanding.

Our brain stores and organises our sensory experiences so that we can function without having to learn anew each day. It's no good just remembering previous stimuli, they have to be categorised as well; you need a broad understanding of what a door handle does, otherwise every time you encountered one that didn't look quite the same, you'd be trapped in the room while you worked it out.

Similarly with our concepts of 'chair' or 'table', or 'hot', or 'sharp'. Throughout our lives we build on these representations to expand our understanding of the world and our ability to operate within it. Using all our senses is crucial to this. Indeed, according to Professor Vilyanur

astonishing animal abilities

If you think that our human senses are amazing, just look at the sensory capabilities of some other creatures.

- A buzzard can spot a mouse from a height of 4,500m (15,000ft). A falcon can see sharp images even when diving at 100 miles per hour.
- A male silkworm moth can detect the smell of a female moth up to 11 kilometres away.
- An earthworm's entire body is covered with taste receptors.
- Fish and turtles can distinguish the smell of the stream or beach where they were born and use this to navigate.
- Worker honeybees have a ring of iron oxide in their abdomens, which is thought to help them navigate by detecting the Earth's magnetic field.
- Bloodhounds' noses have an odour-detecting area 50 times the size of that of humans and a million times more sensitive. They can follow a scent trail that is nearly four days old.
- Butterflies have hairs on their wings that sense changes in air pressure.
- A dragonfly's eye contains 30,000 lenses.
- Some sharks can detect fish extracts in concentrations lower than one part in 10 billion.
- Pit-vipers have a heat-sensitive organ between their eyes and nostrils to help them track down prey, even in the dark. It can distinguish temperature changes as tiny as 0.002 to 0.003°C.

Ramachandran, director of the Center for Brain and Cognition at the University of California, San Diego: 'Intersensory interaction is what paved the way for higher intelligence capacity in humans.'

Our senses also keep us safe. When we experience something outside those familiar categories, something that doesn't compute, our brain and our senses go into a state of high alert, to prepare us for the unexpected. They are especially attuned to detect change, because it may spell danger.

LIFE-ENHANCING

And, essentially, our senses are also hard-wired into the pleasure centres of our brain – we are supposed to enjoy life. That's what drives us to eat, drink, hug, fall in love, have sex and even exercise.

All these activities promote the release of chemicals in the brain that make us feel happy, satisfied and rewarded. We are biologically programmed to seek them out because they are crucial to our survival, individually and as a species. So enjoying your senses is what life's all about.

That's why your *Smart Sense Plan* isn't just about preserving useful functions; it's also about adding spice to life, relishing the joy that our senses give us and preserving that pleasure ... for life.

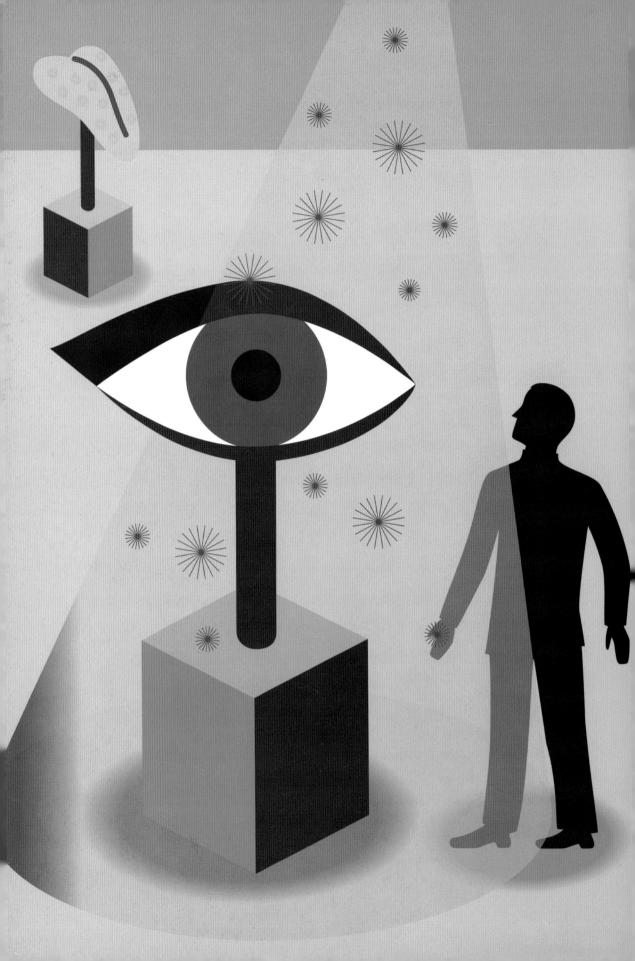

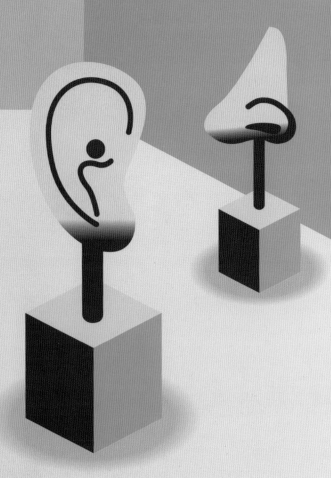

Sight

Your eyes are one of your most precious assets. Discover how they work, what steps you should take to protect your sight, and how to develop a **Smart Sense Plan** to preserve your vision for life. Find out about inevitable changes that occur as we age, the potential problems and – crucially – what **you** can do, and what the latest medical advances can achieve.

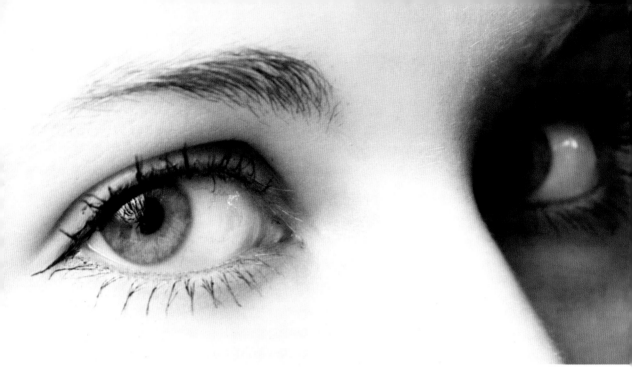

1   The miracle of sight

Every day the papers bombard us with health advice – 'lose weight!', 'take more exercise'; 'cut down on salt, beer, butter, coffee, sugar ...'. The messages urging us to safeguard our health are everywhere. But how often are you told to look after your eyes?

We should all value them more. Sight underpins our mobility, our safety and our independence – and it gives us huge enjoyment from simple things, such as reading a book, to lifelong pleasures, such as watching children and grandchildren change and grow. Yet thousands of people in Britain lose their sight needlessly, even though lifestyle changes and regular eye tests could save it or at least minimise the damage.

TAKEN FOR GRANTED

As children and young adults, many of us take our eyes for granted. We can read distant signs, notices, even the small print on credit agreements with ease and can't imagine not being able to do so. We get impatient with our parents when they can't find their glasses or ask us to thread a needle. But in middle age, something irritating begins to happen. Printed words

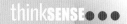

may start to look fuzzy, we have to hold the newspaper at arm's length and we find driving at night increasingly uncomfortable. We gradually realise that our eyes – these wonderfully complex structures – are not infallible.

Because changes tend to happen gradually, many people aren't aware of them – and others are unwilling to admit that their sight is deteriorating. In one UK study at Warwick University, testing people with no apparent sight problems, one in three failed a basic eye chart test – and 65 per cent of those who failed were drivers. A third of those who failed confessed that they had suspected that their eyesight wasn't perfect.

Research by the UK's Royal National Institute of Blind People (RNIB) showed that a third of all drivers in Britain do not have regular eye tests – which means that as many as 13 million people are potentially endangering themselves and others by driving with poor eyesight – and possibly breaking the law and invalidating their insurance as well. In chapter 5, you'll learn what precautions to take when driving and learn plenty of *Smart Sense* strategies to compensate for almost all eyesight changes.

WOULD YOUR EYES PASS A ROAD TEST?

The legal requirement for driving in the UK is that you can read a number plate on a stationary car from 20 metres – that's about five cars' length away. If you need glasses or contact lenses to do so, you must wear them while driving. This is particularly important as you get older. In one study, the National Research Council in the USA found that 40 per cent of drivers aged 65 to 74 had difficulty seeing many road signs at the standard distances. Declining vision may be one reason why car accidents are the most common cause of accidental death in this age group, and people over 65 have more accidents per mile driven than any other group except teenagers.

LOOKING AFTER YOUR EYES

As you start to follow the *Smart Sense Plan*, you'll learn to Protect your sight, Assess it, Correct as necessary and generally Enjoy the joys of clear vision – the PACE strategy that runs through this book. Then, you'll be safer, not just on the road, but everywhere. Worsening eyesight, for instance, is often to blame for falls that cause fractures in older people – jeopardising their independence. You'll discover what you can do to minimise the dangers in chapter 5.

You'll also learn how to spot potential sight problems in advance and, in some cases, prevent them. If things do go wrong, this book outlines how to deal with them effectively or compensate for them. The following chapters include information, tools, questionnaires and practical performance tests to help you to assess your sight. But the first important step is up to you; having your eyesight tested regularly by a professional.

ACT PROMPTLY IF YOUR EYESIGHT CHANGES

Deteriorating eyesight may be an inevitable consequence of ageing, but there are easy ways to compensate. An inexpensive measure, such as buying a pair of reading glasses, solves the inconvenience and irritation of not being able to read the newspaper report below the headlines, the cooking instructions on packaged food, or the dosage on a prescription. And if you have more serious problems, there are often effective treatments. Failing to seek help could mean that your eyesight deteriorates more than it needs to.

NEVER MISS AN EYE TEST

Too many people wait for something to go wrong with their vision before doing anything to look after it. The first step is to be aware of your starting point: just how good – or bad – is your eyesight right now?

As the Warwick study shows, all too many of us have no idea. According to the RNIB, more than 200,000 people in the UK have severely impaired vision – when regular eye tests could have saved their sight. This sad statistic reinforces the importance of eye tests, so that disorders such as glaucoma, which is often symptomless, can be detected early; glaucoma is the UK's leading cause of preventable blindness and the second leading cause worldwide, after cataracts.

So if you haven't had an eye test within the past two years, why not book one straightaway? If anything is wrong, you need to know and act quickly for the best chance of effective treatment. Just as importantly, eye tests can detect changes that signal serious health problems, such as diabetes, high blood pressure or raised cholesterol. So think of your eye test as a potential life-saver, rather than just a vision check.

According to the RNIB, more than 200,000 people in the UK have severely impaired vision – when regular eye tests could have saved their sight.

HEALTHY BODY, HEALTHY EYES

In the chapters that follow, you will learn how to maintain, preserve and even enhance your eyesight, developing a personal strategy for life-long good vision.

Chapter 2 explains how to protect your sight, and what risk factors – including family traits, your health, your environment or lifestyle – could influence the quality of your vision. The eye, which is part of the brain, is a highly sophisticated organ – but it's also fragile and easily damaged. You will also discover what you need to do to look after your sight, protect

EYE EMERGENCIES

Just occasionally, eye problems simply cannot wait. Seek immediate, urgent advice from a doctor or eye hospital for any eye injury, including a scratch or burn, or any object embedded in or stuck to the front of your eye. If you get a chemical in your eye, wash it out thoroughly with water first but see a doctor as soon as possible.

Other eye emergencies include sudden complete or partial loss of vision in one or both eyes, or sudden persistent or severe pain in or around the eye. You should seek help if you become extremely sensitive to light, see halos or rainbow effects around lights, suffer blurred vision or double vision that lasts more than a few minutes, or the sudden appearance of flashes, black spots or large batches of 'floaters'. Severe redness, itching, burning or excessive watering of the eye, or a profuse greenish or white discharge from the eye are also symptoms that require immediate attention.

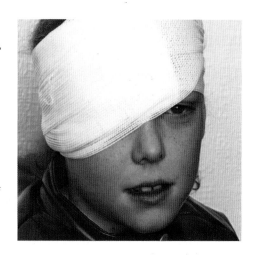

your eyes against injury and against hazardous environmental factors, including sunlight or computer glare and strain. A healthy lifestyle is as important for your eyes as it is for your body, so you will find out which foods can help to enhance your vision and protect against eye disease – and which you should avoid. You'll discover why smoking and obesity are bad for your eyes as well as your body, and why exercise is good for your eyes as well as your waistline.

CHOICES, CHOICES

Another important part of your *Smart Sense Plan* is to assess your sight and take corrective action if necessary. Chapter 3 outlines in greater detail all the things that an eye test can detect; once you know the current state of your sight, you'll be alert to any changes and you'll be able to spot problems early (See the panel, above, for eye emergencies.) In the following chapters you'll discover a wealth of information and advice on self-help measures as well as options for improving your sight, and the most effective treatments for conditions that need professional help.

Sometimes the choices can be confusing – should you try glasses or contact lenses? What sort of lenses are best for you? Would laser surgery be suitable for your sight problems? What's the best option if you develop cataracts? This book will guide you through the many possibilities and give expert views on what does and doesn't work, and what you can hope for from future developments.

With your *Smart Sense Plan* in place, you will have all the tools you need to ensure that you have the best chance to preserve your sight and remain self-reliant, perform well at work, enjoy your hobbies and find sheer joie de vivre – for the rest of your life!

how the eye works

The eye works in much the same way as a camera; the eye detects incoming light reflected from objects in our environment and transforms it into images. At the back of the eye, a delicate, light-sensitive tissue called the retina, which is only about the thickness of a piece of paper, senses these images, similar to the film in a camera, then sends them to the laboratory – in this case, your brain – for processing into 'pictures' of the outside world.

As the light travels into the eye, it has to be focused so that it creates an accurate image. This involves bending or 'refracting' the light rays inwards, so that they reach a point at which a clear image is formed. In people with perfect vision, this 'focal point' is exactly on the retina – if not, the image will be blurred, which is what happens if you are short-sighted or long-sighted.

making pictures

1 Light travels to the eye from a distant object (the flower) in parallel rays.

2 The eye's lens bends the light rays inwards, making them converge on a spot called the fovea centralis which is within the macula lutea on the retina.

3 This results in an upside-down image on the retina. Also, light reflected by one side of an object is reflected on the opposite side of the retina, producing a mirror image on the retina.

4 Impulses created by the image on the retina are sent down the optic nerve to the brain, where they are processed into an image of the object that is 'seen' the right way up.

Parallel light rays are bent (refracted) when they pass through any substance; therefore light is refracted as it passes through layers of the eye. Unlike the other layers of the eye, the lens has the ability to change its shape and so alter the degree to which it refracts light.

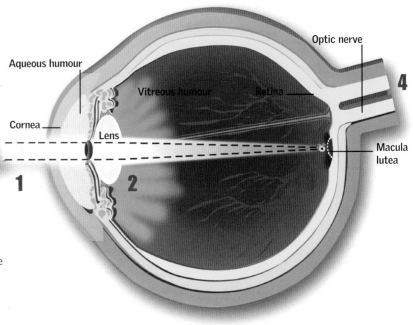

Optic nerve

Aqueous humour

Vitreous humour

Retina

4

Cornea

Lens

Macula lutea

1

2

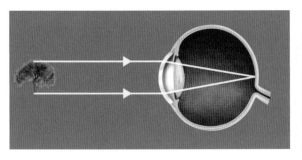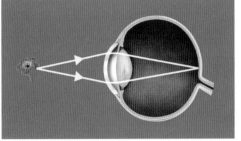

The eye's lens is extremely flexible – particularly when we are young. This means that it can change shape easily to focus on distant objects and then refocus on something that is close-up. As we get older the lens becomes stiffer and refocusing takes longer.

PICTURE PERFECT

Light rays are actually bent twice as they pass into the eye. Most refraction takes place at the cornea, a transparent but tough covering that sits over the iris (the coloured ring) and pupil (the black circle in the middle of the iris) like a casing on a watch, to protect the eye while allowing light through. Problems arise if the cornea bends the light rays too much, causing short-sightedness, or not enough, leading to long-sightedness – and chapter 3 explains more about these common sight conditions.

Next, light rays are bent in again as they pass through the lens, which sits directly behind the pupil. To form an accurate image, light from nearby objects needs bending more than that from far away objects – meaning that the eye must change its focus, or 'accommodate' from distant to near vision. Unlike a camera lens, the lens of the eye is flexible, relaxing and contracting to become thicker or thinner and so change its strength, enabling the eye to focus on both distant and near objects.

DON'T LET FLOATERS ALARM YOU

'Floaters' are semi-transparent spots, blobs or cobweb-like threads that may drift across your field of vision and move around as you move your eyes. They are due to stray fibres and cellular debris trapped in the normally transparent, jelly-like substance called vitreous humour that fills the larger cavity of the eyeball, behind the lens (see diagram, left). As they float by, they cast a shadow on the retina, and it's the shadow that makes you aware of them, especially if you're looking at a plain background, such as a pale wall or a clear sky.

Most people have a few floaters and they get more common as the vitreous humour liquefies and shrinks slightly, especially after the age of 50. Short-sighted people and diabetics may have more floaters earlier in life, and they can increase after cataract operations, laser eye surgery or an eye

FLOATING WARNING

Usually floaters increase in number gradually. Very rarely a sudden new batch of floaters may signal some other eye problem, especially if accompanied by flashing lights or loss of vision at the periphery (what you see out of the corner of your eye). Report such symptoms to a doctor or optician at once, as this can occur with a complication of diabetes called diabetic retinopathy, or with retinal detachment that needs immediate treatment to prevent blindness.

injury. In most cases, floaters are harmless. Yet, interestingly, this is a symptom that patients often report to their doctors or eye specialists. In one UK survey in South Derbyshire, opticians said that they each saw on average 14 patients a month who were concerned about floaters.

If you've never noticed them before, or if they're increasing in size or quantity, they can be alarming and bothersome. In some cases, looking rapidly up and down will encourage them to move out of your field of vision. Floaters usually settle within a few months and they become less noticeable as your brain learns to ignore them.

your remarkable retina

The retina, at the back of your eye, contains photoreceptor cells that respond to light. There are two types of cells – rods and cones. Rods are extremely sensitive and need very little light to function. In a cinema, we use our cones to see the screen and our rods to find a seat. Rods are also brilliant for detecting movement. A cat has a rod-based retina that it uses, for instance, to detect a mouse scampering in undergrowth at twilight. Rods contain only one type of light-sensitive pigment (the rod image is black and white, with shades of grey) and aren't used for colour vision.

Cones give us fine detailed colour vision and are good at dealing with rapidly changing images, but they need considerable light to function properly. Based on pigment content, there are three types of cones, usually called blue, green and red (the wavelength of the light they can best detect). Working in concert, the three sets of cones give us a complex visual balance, which the brain interprets as colour and hue. There are about 120 million rods and 6 million cones in the human retina.

THE HUB OF THE EYE

An especially sensitive area called the macula lutea lies at the centre of the retina. Here, in an eye with normal sight, incoming light rays are focused. Only this little area – around 5.5mm wide – allows us really detailed vision, which is why we need to turn our eyes towards printed text or look directly at people's faces, in order to focus on them properly; you can't read a book or recognise a face out of the corner of your eye.

In the centre of the macula is a small pit, called the fovea, which has an especially high concentration of cones, enabling us to see straight ahead, appreciate subtle shades of colour and distinguish fine detail.

FEAST YOUR EYES

The macula is also called the 'yellow spot' because of its high concentration of yellow-orange pigments – these are the same pigments that are found in some fruit and vegetables.

Research suggests that this colour link is more than superficial. Ensuring a good intake of fruit, vegetables and other nutrients should be part of everyone's *Smart Sense Plan* because such a diet can actually help you to safeguard the health of your macula and protect against sight-threatening eye diseases. Later on (see page 38), you will find out which fruits and vegetables contain most of these pigments and are especially beneficial.

SUPER-VISION

Have you ever wondered why some people have much sharper vision than others? It's because the number, type and distribution of cones in the retina vary between people. The more densely packed your cones are within the macula, the more acute your vision will be, because more cones react to incoming light and more signals are sent to the brain giving more information about the scene viewed and consequently better-than-normal eyesight. But – unless colour blind – everyone perceives colour in the same way; while the eyes have colour-sensitive receptors, colour interpretation is a function of the brain.

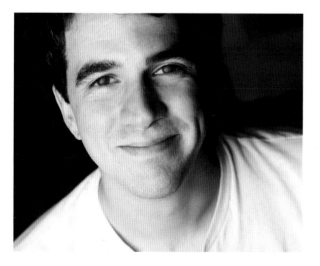

'Red-eye' – diagnosis and cure

The devilish red gleam in photographs is due to light reflected back from the blood vessels supplying the retina. It occurs when the pupil cannot contract quickly enough to stop the light bouncing back into the camera lens. The cure is to position the flash to the side or above the camera or to bounce light off a nearby white surface, as professional photographers do. If you have a built-in flash, try asking your subjects to look over your shoulder. Most new cameras include a red-eye reduction setting, which fires a series of pre-flashes, causing the pupils to contract before the final flash.

night vision

WHY IT GETS HARDER TO SEE IN THE DARK

Rods – the photoreceptor cells in the retina responsible for night vision – are concentrated around the periphery of the retina. Over the course of a lifetime, most cone cells remain intact, but we lose around a third of our rods – which is why it gets harder to see in the dark as we get older. Our rods also take longer to adjust when moving from bright to dimmer light and we become less good at spotting movements out of the corners of our eyes – the periphery of our visual field.

PUPIL POWER

Just like a camera aperture setting, your eye can alter the diameter of the pupil to control the amount of light it lets in. In dim light, the pupil gets wider to let in more light. The area of your pupil more than doubles in size in near darkness, and shrinks in very bright light to around half the size it is under normal room lighting. In young eyes, this adjustment happens almost instantaneously; it's a little slower and less efficient in older ones.

The area of your pupil more than doubles in size in near darkness, and shrinks in very bright light to around half the size it is under normal room lighting.

Changes in pupil size are due to contraction and expansion of the iris, the coloured part of the eye surrounding the pupil, which is actually a ring of muscle. In common with other muscles, it weakens with age, so pupils are less responsive to sudden changes in light level. Our pupils get smaller as we get older; 20-year-olds with a pupil diameter of 4.7mm in daylight can expand this by 3.3mm to around 8mm when they go into a dark room; by contrast 70-year-olds can add just 0.5mm to their average daylight pupil size of 2.7mm. This means that their pupils, at their night-time best, are just 3.2mm wide – less than what 20-year-olds enjoy in daylight – rather like asking the youngsters to wear sunglasses in the dark.

NIGHT DRIVING

Fewer rods, smaller pupils – no wonder we find it harder to drive at night as we get older. In fact, a 50-year-old needs roughly twice as much light to see as well as a 30-year-old after dark, and is less able to adapt to a sudden increase in brightness, such as the glare of oncoming car headlights. Don't worry, though – there are ways you can combat these irritating changes, such as eating foods that help to improve night sight, as well as strategies to prepare for – and even enjoy – night driving (see pages 106-107).

the **colour** question

The colour of your iris depends on the amount and type of pigment present. This pigment is vital to sight, as it blocks light transmission through the iris itself. A transparent iris simply would not work, as it would let far too much light into the eye. That's one reason why albinos, who have a genetic pigment disorder, tend to have poor eyesight.

Whether you have blue, green, hazel or brown eyes may seem purely cosmetic, but some evidence suggests that the colour of your eyes could indicate possible health risks. For example, psychologists at Georgia State University in Atlanta found that people with light-coloured eyes were more likely than dark-eyed individuals to abuse alcohol. It seems dark-eyed people have a greater sensitivity to alcohol that prevents them from drinking the large quantities necessary to produce physical dependence.

So if you have light eyes – green, blue, grey or hazel – rather than brown – it might be a good idea to watch your alcohol intake. But people with brown eyes are not immune, research also suggests that they are more prone to cataracts and high blood pressure than people with light eyes.

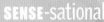
SENSE-sational

LOOK INTO MY EYES

The idea that our eyes reveal our character is nonsense, isn't it? Not necessarily, say behavioural scientists from Sweden's Örebro University and Karolinska Institute. They tested the personality characteristics of 428 students and matched them to their iris patterns. They report in the journal *Biological Psychology* that students who were warm, trusting and empathic had more dense iris crypts, the wavy lines that radiate out from the pupil. In contrast, furrows in the iris – curved lines that form around the outer edge when the pupils dilate and contract – were more numerous and extended further in students who tested high for impulsiveness.

During foetal growth, the researchers say, certain genes that influence the parts of the brain involved with emotion and response to rewards, also affect iris patterns, suggesting a link between iris patterns and specific personality traits.

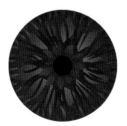
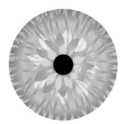
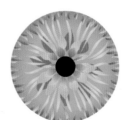
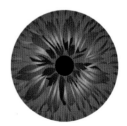

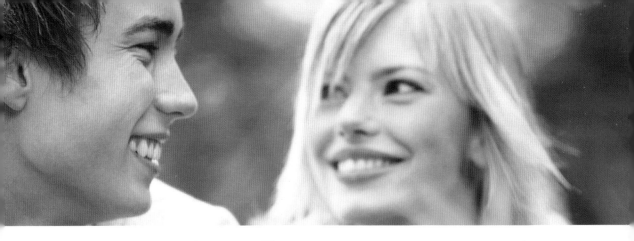

the look of love

Pupil size is affected by emotions as well as by light levels. If you are angry or you see something disgusting, the pupil gets narrower or contracts. If you look at someone you love, or something delicious to eat, it expands, or 'dilates'.

Pupil dilation is a proven measure of interest and attraction. In one classic study, men were shown photographs of women that had been artificially retouched to make the pupils appear either larger or smaller. The men invariably found the women with larger pupils more attractive and friendlier than the same women with smaller pupils, though none of them were consciously aware why they made this choice.

... or fear

There is an exception to the general rule that positive feelings make the pupils dilate and negative ones make them contract – fear. A frightened person will often have widely-dilated pupils, because fear creates a rush of the stress hormone adrenaline, in preparation for a primitive 'fight or flight' response; that response includes pupil dilation to improve visual sensitivity.

... or empathy

We use pupil changes in assessing other people's emotions, though we are usually not consciously aware of the subtle differences in pupil size. What's more, our own pupils react in response – in one study at University College London, volunteers who looked at pictures of sad faces with small pupils showed a corresponding reduction in their own pupil size. Such reactions may be important in the development of empathy. Scientists already know that when we feel in tune with someone we tend to mimic their posture and movements. It seems that body language mimicry starts with the eyes.

testing, testing

There are many good reasons for having regular eye tests, from feeling comfortable when reading or watching TV to saving your sight – for life.

As we get older, the lens of the eye, and the tiny muscles that control it, get less efficient at altering its focus. That's why almost everyone, sooner or later, starts to have difficulty focusing on objects close up. This common condition, known medically as presbyopia, is easily remedied with reading glasses.

GLAUCOMA - DON'T RISK IT

Anyone over 40 is also at increased risk of glaucoma – a leading cause of blindess in the UK. This eye condition is easily detected with a simple eye test and usually quite treatable, but can cause sight loss if not promptly spotted and dealt with. Glaucoma occurs because of damage to the optic nerve that carries signals from the retina to the brain.

The lens effectively divides the eyeball into two parts or chambers. The tiny anterior chamber in front of the lens is filled with a clear fluid, called aqueous humour, which is continually produced within the eye. Therefore it needs to drain away again, and any obstruction to drainage raises the internal pressure within the eyeball. This raised pressure can lead to glaucoma, which may cause few initial symptoms but, left untreated, can permanently damage vision, which is why regular eye testing is so important. You will learn more about glaucoma in chapter 4.

DAMAGE LIMITATION

One of the main causes of sight loss in people over 50 affects the retina. Known as age-related macular degeneration (AMD), this progressive disease damages the macula lutea, the tiny area at the centre of the retina, which enables us to see fine detail. Regular eye testing will also ensure that early signs of this potentially devastating condition are spotted – and, again, you can start taking action to fight it.

Another problem that gets more common with age is clouding of the lens, known as cataract. Cataracts are the world's leading cause of blindness – but again they can be easily and successfully treated. In the following chapters you'll find out who's at risk, and discover some simple things you can do to protect your eyes from cataracts. You'll also learn how to spot the signs of a developing cataract, so that you can seek treatment when necessary.

refreshing tears

When exposed to the air, our eyes need protection. A thin transparent membrane called the conjunctiva, which covers the white of the eye and lines the upper and lower lids, stops the eyes from drying out. Tiny glands called lacrimal glands beneath the upper, outer corner of each eyelid continually secrete a watery tear fluid that is spread over the eye surface every time we blink, maintaining a constant moist layer and preventing damage from tiny particles in the air.

In addition, even smaller glands called meibomian glands at the inner edge of the eyelids themselves add an oily, lipid secretion that lubricates the eye and reduces evaporation of tear fluid.

PROTECTIVE TEARS

As well as the constant tear film that keeps our eyes moist, we produce excess tear fluid when we need to wash out irritants, such as specks of dust, or in response to injury, infection or allergies.

The composition of these free-flowing tears is chemically different to the normal basal tear film – they contain more of an enzyme called lysozyme, a natural antibacterial substance that helps to counteract infection. The concentration of lysozyme in tears tends to be low in children, increases until middle age and then falls off again, which may be why children and older people are more susceptible to eye infections.

As we get older, tear production is often reduced and the tear film contains less of the oils needed to keep it from drying out – which may result in dry eye syndrome. This can make night driving difficult, as symptoms include a gritty sensation in the eyes, blurriness of vision and a dislike of bright lights.

BRIGHTER OUTLOOK

But, for all these problems, there are practical solutions, as you'll discover in the following chapters. You'll find out more about your eyes and how to take care of them, helping you to develop your personal *Smart Sense Plan* for enjoying the miracle of sight – for life.

SENSE-sational

HEALING POWER

Crying can do you a world of good – and perhaps not just as an emotional release. Researchers have discovered that tears shed in extreme emotional situations have a higher protein content and more manganese and prolactin than ordinary tears or than those produced, for instance, in response to peeling an onion. As we produce more manganese and prolactin when we're stressed, some scientists now believe that emotional tears may help to eliminate these and other toxic stress-related chemicals.

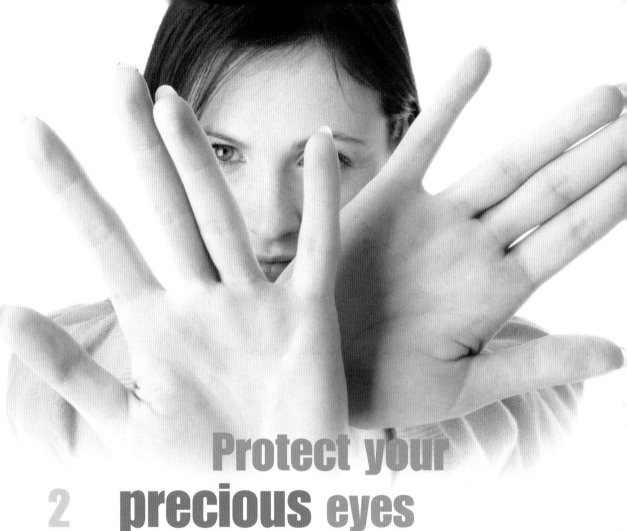

Protect your
2 precious eyes

The human body is a remarkable machine. But like any other machine, parts of it can break down if we don't look after it. The eyes are a prime example. We don't even consider them until something goes wrong.

This chapter will explain how aspects of everyday living can damage your sight and what steps you can take to protect it, both by adjusting what happens on the outside, and also by looking after what happens inside. Did you know, for instance, that being overweight is a risk factor? According to the Royal National Institute of Blind People (RNIB), Britain's 10 million obese adults and 2 million obese children run twice the risk of losing their sight prematurely as a result of developing diabetes or age-related macular degeration (AMD), which has also been linked to obesity. If your eyesight has begun to deteriorate, you will discover how to slow or stop the decline – or even to reverse the trend.

light matters

The first thing to remember is that bright sunlight can harm your vision. It increases damage from free radical formation in the eye and, according to the American Academy of Ophthalmology, long hours in direct sun can damage your eyes and contribute to cataracts and macular degeneration. Ultraviolet and blue light cause most damage over long periods, so it makes sense to put on a broad-brimmed hat and a pair of sunglasses, along with the suncream. Reflected light is equally dangerous. Humans evolved in an unreflective environment of earth and trees. Concrete pavements and modern buildings reflect far more light, making us more vulnerable to light damage. It's also important to protect your eyes when on sand, water or snow which reflect very efficiently.

BLURRING THE DIFFERENCE

While sunlight can cause damage, so can working long hours inside under fluorescent office lighting. We spend much of our daily lives under artificial light – which may contribute to short sight, as you'll discover in the next chapter. This runs counter to our nature; human eyes evolved to spend daylight hours outdoors and nights in near-total darkness.

Unlike our distant ancestors, who slept a lot longer during winter nights, we spend many hours of darkness under artificial light. Often we sleep in rooms that let in outside light, which can adversely affect our eyes, as eyes need darkness to rest effectively.

STOP FEELING 'SAD'

Natural light and darkness help to set our body clock. Any disruption, such as jet lag or shift work, can upset the rhythm. This is because the region in our brain that controls the timing of many biological functions – such as when we feel hungry or sleepy – is 'set' by light-dark cycles.

Until recently, scientists thought that the signals for these 'circadian rhythms' came from the rods and cones of the retina (see page 24). But recent research has shown that they are actually sent from another type of specialised cell in the retina – called a ganglion cell. These cells specifically

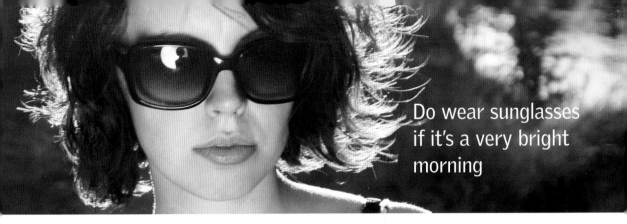

Do wear sunglasses if it's a very bright morning

detect sky-blue light, and 'turn on' at about the same intensity as the daylight at dawn. Without this specific 'switch on' signal, we are vulnerable to insomnia, fatigue and mood disturbances, including the winter depression, known as SAD (seasonal affective disorder) that affects many people living in northern climates.

BOOST THE CONTRAST

The more contrast you can maintain between night and daylight levels, the better you sleep and the better it is for your eyes, it seems. If there's a streetlight outside your bedroom window, hang thicker curtains or black-out blinds. During daylight hours, spend more time outdoors. Get out of doors at weekends as well, and position furniture in the house so that you get more natural daylight in the places where you spend most time.

everyday eye care

Our eyes are also not designed to cope with prolonged close work – whether reading or working at a computer screen. It can cause eyestrain, which may not do permanent damage but can make eyes feel gritty and uncomfortable, or cause a headache and blurred vision. (In the next chapter you'll discover why scientists are also linking close work to worldwide increases in shortsightedness.) There are some simple, immediate steps you can take to lessen eyestrain when doing close work.

● Glance up briefly at regular intervals – look away for a second or so, perhaps, at the end of every page. Move your eyes from side to side, or gaze at a distant object, to break the intense focus on one near point.

● Every 30 to 45 minutes have a complete change of scenery – take a 3 to 5 minute break to do something in a completely different environment, such as making a cup of tea or having a brief stroll outside.

● Wear glasses if you need them for close work, so that your eyes don't have to work so hard – and keep your prescription up to date.

SCREEN JUNKIES

There are several reasons why computer work causes eyestrain. What we do on our computers – whether playing games or working on computer-aided design (CAD) – involves intense, focused concentration. We tend to spend longer periods at the computer than we would, say, reading a book. And our blink rate is often reduced during computer use. All this can cause dry eyes, blurring and eyestrain, plus other complaints such as neck, shoulder and wrist pain, or headaches.

WHAT'S THE DAMAGE?

Until recently, most scientists said that spending so much time in front of a computer might make your eyes tired, but it wouldn't damage them. But a 2004 study in Japan suggested that there are possibly other dangers.

Researchers from Toho University School of Medicine in Tokyo assessed nearly 10,000 Japanese workers from four different companies, asking them about computer use at home and at work, and any history of eye disease. They found that heavy use of computers was often associated with long or shortsightedness. What's more, in tests, about one in three of these workers had suspected glaucoma.

Statistical analysis suggested that heavy computer use, glaucoma and short-sightedness (myopia) were interlinked. The team speculates that short-sighted eyes may be more susceptible to eyestrain from prolonged computer use. As Japanese people are prone to short sightedness and also to a particular form of glaucoma (chronic closed angle), it is not clear whether these results necessarily apply to other populations.

But many eye specialists are cautious. David Wright, chief executive of the International Glaucoma Association advises heavy computer users to have regular comprehensive eye tests 'to detect the earliest possible signs of glaucoma when treatment is most effective'. In the UK, computer users are entitled to a free eye test paid for by their employers.

think**SENSE** ● ● ●

THE IMPORTANCE OF BLINKING

People tend to blink less when using a computer. When you blink, your eyelids operate a bit like windscreen wipers, spreading tear film over the surface of the eye to keep it moist, and sweeping away dust and dirt particles. Although you can blink voluntarily, it usually happens unconsciously, on average around 13 times a minute – about once every 4 to 5 seconds. When you look downwards, your eyelid covers more of your eye surface, and you tend to blink more often – so having your screen below eye level and tilted back will reduce the tendency to a wide-eyed, fixed stare and help to ensure that your eyes are kept moist.

SAFETY FIRST

Another danger when working at the computer is that we stare and forget to blink (see box, left). Blinking is the eye's natural defence mechanism against injury. If anything gets too close to the eye, the lid will close – an involuntary reflex that is almost impossible to control. But your eyelids are quite thin and fragile. Sometimes extra protection is essential.

Experts reckon that at least 90 per cent of eye injuries could be avoided. At work, for example, about 70 per cent of eye injuries are caused by flying or falling objects, or sparks – and more than one in ten will cause temporary or permanent loss of vision. But a shocking three-fifths of people injured are either not wearing eye protection at the time of the accident, or wearing the wrong type. Many eye accidents occur in the 'safe' home environment where people often take unnecessary risks – the welder who uses a mask at work but forgets to when working on his car.

A shocking three-fifths of people injured are either not wearing eye protection at the time of the accident, or wearing the wrong type.

Common causes of eye injury include DIY, gardening, work, sport and traffic accidents. You can't always tell how much damage has been done, so you should always have an injured eye examined by a doctor even if the injury seems trivial.

Follow the guidelines below to minimise your risk.

- If eye protection is recommended for an activity, wear it. Ordinary glasses don't always give adequate protection – and hard lenses and spectacles can also cause severe eye injuries if they shatter on impact.
- Always follow your employer's safety recommendations if your work involves any kind of risk to your eyes.
- Use safety goggles for home DIY, and keep tools in good condition.
- If you play sports regularly, especially racquet sports such as squash, ask your optician about polycarbonate sports glasses or goggles (this is the material used in plastic riot shields and military aircraft canopies – it can withstand the force of a .22 calibre bullet).
- Follow the safety instructions on power tools to the letter, and handle all chemicals – including household cleaning products – with care.
- Inspect your lawn for stones, gravel, loose bits of wood and other debris before mowing.

Continued on p38 ➤

an eye-friendly
workstation

In this new age of computer technology, the internet is, for many of us, another window on the world. It's such an integral part of many of our lives, that we pay scant attention to potential eye risks. To minimise eye strain, set up your computer as shown below and follow the guidelines on the opposite page.

ARE YOU SITTING COMFORTABLY?

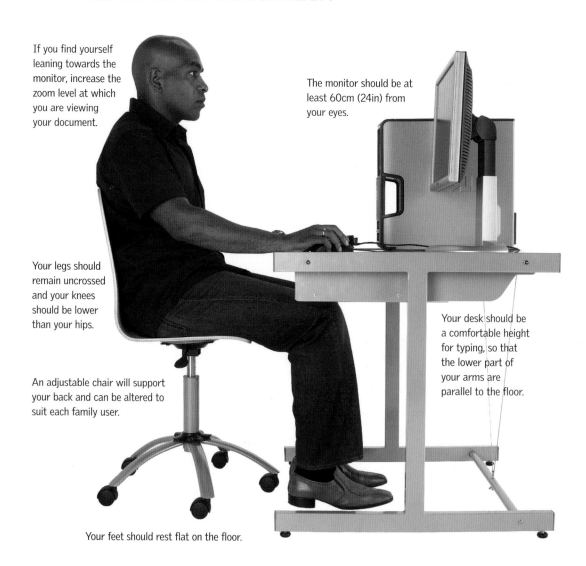

If you find yourself leaning towards the monitor, increase the zoom level at which you are viewing your document.

The monitor should be at least 60cm (24in) from your eyes.

Your legs should remain uncrossed and your knees should be lower than your hips.

Your desk should be a comfortable height for typing, so that the lower part of your arms are parallel to the floor.

An adjustable chair will support your back and can be altered to suit each family user.

Your feet should rest flat on the floor.

GUIDELINES FOR EYE-SAFE WORKING

- Don't sit too close to your screen – position it at least 60cm (24in) from your eyes
- If you can't read comfortably at this distance, increase the size of the text rather than getting closer to the screen.
- Position your screen so that you are looking downwards at it; modern lightweight flat screens are much easier to adjust than the older heavy ones.
- If possible tilt the top part of the screen slightly backwards. This is a more natural position for your eyes than a vertical screen (think of how you read a book or magazine).
- Use indirect lighting where possible, from above or to the side of the screen, not behind or in front of it.
- Minimise reflected glare from lights or windows – if some glare is unavoidable, you could fit a glare filter over the screen.
- Keep your screen clean and dust-free.
- When taking vision breaks, don't read a book or catch up on your post. Instead try to do something that does not involve focusing close up – get up and walk around, look out of the window, take out the rubbish or potter in the garden.

self-test questionnaire
Are you at risk?

Are you shortsighted? Do you regularly use a computer? Here's a simple test to discover if you may be at increased risk of glaucoma. First, find your scores in questions 1 and 2.

1 How many years have you been using a computer?

- ☐ 0-5   (score 1 point)
- ☐ 5-10   (score 2 points)
- ☐ 10-20 (score 3 points)
- ☐ 20-plus (score 4 points)

2 How may hours a day on average do you spend on the computer

- ☐ 0-1   (score 1 point)
- ☐ 1-4   (score 2 points)
- ☐ 4-8   (score 3 points)
- ☐ 8-plus (score 4 points)

Now multiply your two scores to find out your user level:

A score of 1-3 indicates light use; 4-8 is moderate use; 9-16 is heavy use.

Light users run no increased risk of glaucoma; moderate users may be increasing their risk by more than a third and heavy users, by almost three quarters.

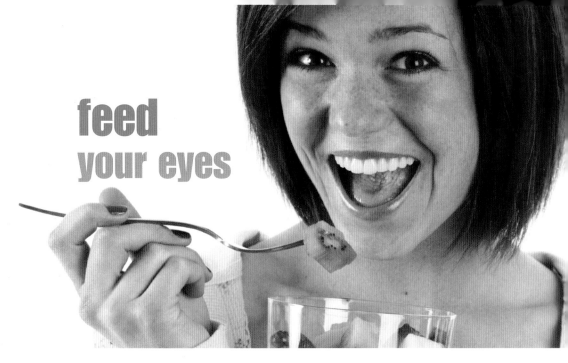

feed your eyes

Did you know that some foods can actually boost your eyesight? Or that certain nutrients are vital for eye health? Read on to find out why your grandmother was right about carrots helping you to see in the dark, and why a sophisticated brunch – Eggs Florentine (poached or baked eggs on a bed of wilted spinach) – is a particularly eye-healthy meal.

GOLD-MEDAL EYE NUTRIENTS

In chapter 1, the macula (the area of the retina that provides most detailed vision) was described as the 'yellow spot'. This is because it is in fact yellow, and the reason is that it contains high levels of two natural plant pigments, lutein and zeaxanthin. These two pigments also make pumpkins look orange and sweetcorn yellow, and they are highly beneficial for your eyes, which is why orange/yellow vegetables and fruits top the list of vision superfoods.

They belong to a group of nutrients called carotenoids, which have powerful antioxidant properties. That means they help to counteract free radicals – highly reactive, and highly damaging, chemicals that form in the body as a result of metabolic processes and exposure to pollutants and radiation. Free radical damage accumulates with age and contributes to eye problems such as age-related macular degeneration (AMD, see page 44). These golden nutrients are also

SENSE-sational

NATURAL SHADES

The lutein pigmentation of the macula absorbs blue ultraviolet (UV) light, the most dangerous wavelength for the eye, so reducing the amount of photo-damage from sunlight. This could help to protect your eyes against both macular degeneration and cataracts. Lutein and other carotenoids have been dubbed 'natural sunglasses'.

found in the lens and seem to protect against cataracts. In a US study of more than 77 thousand female nurses aged 45 to 71 years, women with the highest intakes of lutein and zeaxanthin were 22 per cent less likely than those with the lowest levels to develop cataracts severe enough to require treatment, even after other risk factors such as age and smoking were taken into account. We need to eat five portions of fruit and vegetables a day to stay healthy and lower our risk of eye diseases such as AMD; in the UK, on average, we eat only two.

Good food sources of lutein and zeaxanthin include dark green leafy vegetables such as kale, spinach, Brussels sprouts, cabbage and broccoli, along with sweetcorn, pumpkin, orange peppers, kiwi fruit, red grapes, celery and squash. They are also found in egg yolks. For your eyes' sake, try to include some of these foods in your diet every day.

SEE IN THE DARK WITH BILBERRIES

Sometimes known as European blueberries, bilberries contain blue-red pigments that are also antioxidants. They strengthen capillaries, the tiny blood vessels that deliver nutrients and oxygen to body tissues. They may help to prevent cataracts, and have been shown to increase macular pigmentation, boost retinal blood flow and improve night vision. In fact, during the Second World War, Royal Air Force pilots were encouraged to eat bilberry jam before night missions to improve sight. If you can't get hold of any, try supplements of bilberry extract (160mg twice a day).

A GLASS OF RED WINE A DAY

You probably know that wine – in moderation, of course – is beneficial for your heart; the good news is that it may protect your eyes too. In one major US study of more than 3,000 people aged over 45, a daily glass of wine reduced the risk of developing AMD by around 20 per cent, compared with people who drank beer or spirits or were teetotal. This could be because wine, especially red wine, is high in flavonoids –

ACE superfoods

The following are good sources of these eye-friendly antioxidants:

vitamin A	egg yolks, oily fish and cheese
beta carotene	apricots, carrots, pumpkin, squash, kale, spinach and other green, leafy vegetables
vitamin C	citrus fruits (such as oranges and lemons) and juices, strawberries, kiwi fruits, green peppers, potatoes and dark-green leafy vegetables, such as broccoli
vitamin E	whole grains, vegetable oil, margarine, nuts and seeds
selenium	meat, fish, butter, Brazil nuts, avocados and lentils
zinc	oysters, fish, peanuts and sunflower seeds

think**SENSE** ● ● ●

CARROTS FOR NIGHT SIGHT?

Did Granny get it right? Can carrots really improve your ability to see in the dark? The light sensitive pigment in rod cells – the photoreceptors in the retina responsible for night vision – is partly derived from vitamin A. So foods containing vitamin A, or compounds called carotenoids that are converted to vitamin A in the intestine, are important for eyesight.

Carrots, as their name suggests, are an excellent source of carotenoids. And they are more beneficial cooked than raw. You lose some carotenoid in the cooking but far more is made available for you to absorb because the heat breaks down the cell walls of the vegetable where most of the carotenoids are contained. The same is true of tomatoes.

antioxidants also found in citrus fruits, some vegetables, green tea and cocoa. While wine may help to protect your eyes, not all alcohol is so helpful. Some studies have suggested an increased risk of AMD among beer drinkers.

BRING ON THE KETCHUP

The chief carotenoid in tomatoes is lycopene, which may also help to protect against AMD, as low levels of lycopene have been associated with the development of macular degeneration. Like carrots (see left), they are best cooked to release the lycopene. Rich sources include tomato purée, ketchup and tinned tomatoes.

HAVE A BANANA

If you eat a lot of refined carbohydrates – white bread, white rice and white sugar – at the expense of other nutrients, you could well become chromium-deficient. This mineral helps to strengthen the muscles that control lens focusing, while a chromium deficiency is linked with the development and progression of shortsightedness. Boost your intake of chromium by eating beef, liver, chicken, eggs, wheatgerm, green peppers, apples, bananas, and spinach.

ANTIOXIDANTS FROM A TO ZINC

Many common foods contain powerful antioxidants that may help to protect against eye diseases. According to the Age-Related Eye Disease Study (AREDS), conducted by the National Eye Institute in the USA, antioxidants including beta-carotene, vitamins C and E, zinc and copper, significantly reduced progression of early macular degeneration. Researchers at Tufts University in Boston suggest that vitamins C and E protect against cataracts and slow down their progression. There is also some evidence that vitamin E may slow the progression of short-sightedness in children.

Vitamin A is a constituent of the light-sensitive pigment in retinal cells and is vital for good vision; it is also thought to help cataracts and conjunctivitis. Beta carotene, which is converted to vitamin A in the intestine, has also been found to protect against both macular degeneration and cataracts.

all about fats

Some fats are positively good for your eyes; others can be disastrous. The 'bad' fats – saturated and trans fats – that clog arteries and are linked with heart attacks – are also the fats that are bad for your eyes. Limit your intake by cutting down on red meats and high-fat dairy products such as whole milk, hard cheeses and butter.

Do your utmost to cut down on processed foods, too – cakes, biscuits, crisps, meat pies, take-aways, junk and fast foods. They contain unhealthy trans fats and usually high levels of processed vegetable fats, known as omega-6 fatty acids, which when taken in excess, are known to increase your risk of AMD.

HOW ESSENTIAL?

Omega fatty acids are also known as essential fatty acids (EFAs) because they're vital for many bodily functions including brain, nerve and eyes. Our bodies can't make them: we have to get them from foods.

One type, the omega-3s, are especially good for eyes, helping to reduce inflammation and make the tear film oilier, reducing drying out and alleviating gritty, dry eyes. Research has shown that low omega-3 consumption raises the risk of dry eye syndrome.

To boost eye health, eat two or three portions of oily fish a week, such as sardines, pilchards (fresh or canned), herring and shrimp. Omega-3s are also found in green leafy vegetables, walnuts and some vegetable oils, including flaxseed, rape and soya. You'll do your body a favour, too; these fats are important for the health of your heart, blood vessels and brain.

Our bodies also need some omega-6 fatty acids. These occur in corn oil and many other vegetable oils. But, while we don't eat enough omega-3s, we consume far too many omega-6s in processed and fried foods, which isn't good for eye health.

The ideal ratio of omega-3 to omega-6 is about 1:1 – roughly what our Stone Age ancestors would have consumed. However, in a typical modern diet the ratio is closer to 1:12 (omega-3:omega-6). And if you eat a lot of processed foods, the ratio could be as high as 1:20.

To boost eye health, eat two or three portions of oily fish a week

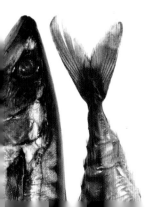
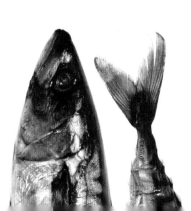
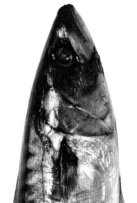
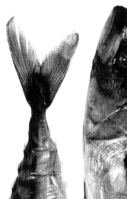

the glycaemic index, or GI

One way to safeguard the long-term health of your eyes – and your heart – is to understand the differences between carbohydrate foods. The 'good' carbohydrates have a low GI; the 'bad' ones have a high GI.

Low GI foods trickle-feed our body systems, producing only small fluctuations in blood sugar and insulin levels. These help to promote weight loss and reduce obesity. High GI foods cause rapidly fluctuating blood sugar levels – a sharp rise after eating, shortly followed by a plummet. That's because the blood sugar surge prompts a corresponding

self-test questionnaire
Are you eating a G-eye diet?

All foods have their own GI rating, with white bread at 100 as the benchmark. When combined with the quantity eaten, this gives a measure of the glycaemic load. But rather than getting out the calculator, the easiest way to improve your diet is simply to swap high-GI foods for low-GI ones. Keep a food diary for the next three days.

Give yourself one point for each portion of low-GI food you eat from this list:

- ☐ Whole grains
- ☐ Fruit
- ☐ Non-starchy vegetables
- ☐ Salad (preferably with vinaigrette dressing)
- ☐ Avocado

- ☐ Legumes (pod vegetables, such as beans and peas)
- ☐ Nuts
- ☐ Seeds
- ☐ Wholemeal bread
- ☐ Brown rice

- ☐ Breakfast cereals based on oats, barley and bran
- ☐ Wholemeal pasta
- ☐ Beef, chicken or fish
- ☐ Eggs

... and deduct one point for each high-GI food from this list:

- ☐ Potatoes
- ☐ White bread
- ☐ White rice

- ☐ Cakes
- ☐ Biscuits
- ☐ Pastries and pies

- ☐ Sweets
- ☐ Crisps
- ☐ Sugary soft drinks

Assuming you're not overeating, an ideal score is between 18 and 25 points over the three days. Add up your score, then swap one food at a time, aiming to increase your score by at least one point a week until you reach the ideal.

If you have access to the internet, you can check the GIs for different foods at www.glycemicindex.com (an online list compiled by the University of Sydney, Australia).

steep rise in insulin, the hormone that enables the body to metabolise sugar. Too much insulin, in turn, causes the sharp drop in blood sugar levels over the next few hours – prompting more carbohydrate cravings. Like sugar, all processed carbohydrates have a high GI, while most fruits have a low GI, causing only a gentle rise and keeping levels more stable.

THE DIABETES CONNECTION

A high intake of refined carbohydrates is already known to increase the risk of diabetes, because repeated demands for insulin, from eating lots of high GI foods, puts a strain on the pancreas where insulin is produced. Both diabetes and obesity can damage your eyesight, but a simple change of diet, that reduces your intake of processed foods, could reduce the risk.

. . . AND SHORTSIGHTEDNESS

Diets high in refined starches, such as breads and cereals, may also be linked to recent dramatic increases in shortsightedness. Bread has been eaten for thousands of years – but not bread as we know it today. Modern refining techniques have hugely increased the rate of starch digestion and, in response, the body pumps out more insulin.

Researchers from Colorado State University in the USA and the University of Sydney in Australia suggest that this could affect children's eye development. If the coordination of eyeball lengthening and lens growth is disturbed during crucial periods, the eyeball may lengthen too much, causing shortsightedness in children. This theory could also help to explain why people who are obese or have adult diabetes are also more likely to become short sighted.

AMD – a disease of civilisation

The condition most likely – on current figures – to rob you of your sight in older age is AMD – age-related macular degeneration. The good news is there is much you can do in earlier life to protect yourself against it.

Scientists now rate AMD – like heart disease and diabetes – a 'disease of civilisation'. What they all have in common are underlying, modern-day risk factors such as high blood pressure, high cholesterol and obesity. In fact the latest research, published in 2008 by the University of Sydney, Australia, has shown that AMD can be used as a pretty accurate predictor of strokes or heart attacks in people aged between 49 and 75 years. The study found that people with early AMD had double the risk of dying from

what about supplements?

For the best eye protection, get your antioxidants from foods rather than supplements, say researchers at the Erasmus Medical Centre in Rotterdam, Holland. But supplements may be helpful in some cases.

B vitamins So many B vitamins are lost during modern food processing that some scientists suggest that people who eat a lot of processed and junk foods should take supplements. And studies by the UK's Medical Research Council show that many older people in Britain are deficient in B vitamins, especially B_{12} and folate. By contrast, people with a high intake of B vitamins, especially folate and riboflavin (B_2), seem to have a reduced risk of cataracts. The Tufts University study (see page 41) also found that women who had higher intakes of two B vitamins – riboflavin and thiamine – had slower cataract progression than women with lower intakes.

Grape seed extract Grape seeds are a rich source of antioxidants – beta carotene, vitamin E and flavonoids. These help to combat free-radical damage in the eye, strengthen the tiny blood vessels (capillaries) of the retina, boost night vision and may protect against cataracts. Some research has suggested that grape seed extract can slow down macular degeneration and perhaps reduce eye strain in people doing a lot of close work.

Rutin Another free radical-busting flavonoid, rutin comes from buckwheat and may help to protect against eye problems such as cataracts and macular degeneration.

Ginkgo biloba Made from the leaves of a Chinese tree fern, ginkgo has long been used in Oriental herbal medicine. It has been reported to improve long-distance visual acuity (detailed vision) in people with AMD. A small study from the University of Brescia in Italy found that 40mg ginkgo three times daily for four weeks also improved the field of vision in some patients with glaucoma.

WHATS the EVIDENCE

CAN SUPPLEMENTS PROTECT YOUR EYESIGHT?

The AREDS study at the US National Eye Institute (see page 41) involved more than 3,500 people aged over 55 in the early stages of AMD. After eight years, those taking antioxidant supplements had about a 28 per cent reduced risk of progressing to advanced AMD and vision loss. These are the doses used in the study:

> vitamin C – 500mg
> vitamin E – 400IU
> beta carotene – 15mg
> zinc (as zinc oxide) – 80mg
> copper (as cupric oxide) – 2mg

The results are highly promising but you should consult your GP or eye specialist before trying the formula. Zinc, for instance, can produce unpleasant side effects on the prostate, and smokers should not take beta carotene as it increases cancer risk.

- Another study looked at the dietary histories of nearly 500 women aged over 50. Those who took daily vitamin C supplements for more than 10 years were 64 per cent less likely to have lens opacities (a sign of cataract).
- Other research has shown that taking 30mg lutein a day increases both blood and retinal levels of this pigment, with a corresponding increase in macular density after five months.

heart disease over the next decade; in those with late AMD the risk jumped five-fold (with the risk of stroke leaping ten-fold). What's behind it? Many of these conditions affect people of normal weight, so it can't be just that we all eat too much. The fact that we eat too many omega-6 fats compared to our intake of omega-3 fats (see page 42) is one possible factor. And modern diets may harbour other dangers.

There are certain things you can do nothing about, such as your age, race and gender as, for instance, white females, aged over 55 are statistically most likely to develop AMD. But look at the other risk factors below to discover how you might lessen your risk and preserve your eyes.

QUIT SMOKING

AMD starts earlier and progresses faster in smokers. Two major British studies have concluded that about a quarter of cases of severe central vision loss from AMD are linked with smoking. The good news is that if you stop (see feature, right), your risk gradually returns to normal.

CUT YOUR FAT INTAKE

On average, we take in about 40 per cent of our food energy as fat. We should be aiming for a healthier level of 20 to 25 per cent. A high-fat diet doesn't just raise your risk of getting AMD, it also increases its severity. In one study at Harvard University involving people over 60 with established AMD, those eating high-fat diets were three times more likely to progress to an advanced form, than those with a low fat intake. And cutting down on 'bad' fats will also help you to avoid another AMD risk factor – obesity.

self-test questionnaire
Risk factors you can remedy

Take the 'smart sense' test below to help you pinpoint any problems – lifestyle and medical – that can be treated and resolved to protect your eyes against AMD.

☐ Do you smoke?　　　　　　　　　　　☐ Do you have high blood pressure?
☐ Is your diet high in fat?　　　　　　　☐ Do you have high cholesterol?
☐ Are you overweight or obese?　　　　☐ Do you have diabetes? (AMD affects nearly
☐ Do you take little or no exercise?　　　40 per cent of diabetics)

If you answer 'yes' to all or any of the questions above, you have some risk of developing AMD as you get older. Read this chapter, talk to your GP and resolve to minimise the risks, one by one.

smoke gets in your eyes

Smoking doubles your risk of sight loss – and if you have a family history of eye disease, the risk may go up eight-fold. If you really can't quit, it's especially important that you do your best to counterbalance its harmful effects by eating an eye-healthy diet (see page 38), though beta carotene supplements, which may heighten cancer risk in smokers, should be avoided.

Remember, though, you are in danger of harming your sight if you continue to smoke. The chemicals in tobacco smoke damage retinal blood vessels and contribute to the development of AMD (see page 44) – it is estimated that about one in ten cases are due to smoking. What's more, the risk of AMD doubles for people who live with smokers – so by giving up cigarettes you are protecting your family, too.

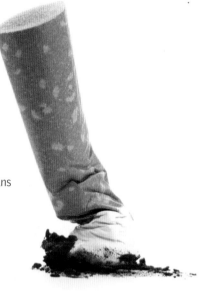

If you do smoke, you risk not only AMD but a host of other eye diseases, including cataracts. If you have health problems such as diabetes or high blood pressure, the chances are that smoking will increase the risk still further.

Get help to stop Most GPs, some pharmacists and even some opticians run clinics to help patients give up smoking – which suggests how important the professionals think it is for your eye health.

You can also telephone the NHS helpline on 0800 169 0169 (open 7 days a week, 7am-11pm) or go to its website at www.gosmokefree.nhs.uk for details of replacement products, local support groups and much more.

your smart sense plan

Your PACE strategy – Protect, Assess, Correct, Enjoy – is beginning to take shape. You've got a good idea of how to Protect your eyesight by taking sensible precautions in your environment. You have strategies to guard against future problems, and you've learnt how to boost your eye health by modifying your diet and lifestyle. If you have written down the aspects that are important to you, this will help you to create a personal plan. You will have started to Assess your sight and may already have had your eyes tested and been fitted with new glasses or lenses.

You don't need to do everything all at once. In fact, it's often better to pick one thing to do at a time – substitute wholemeal bread for your usual white, or resolve to pick up some spinach next time you go shopping – because gradual changes are often the ones that stick. Then, next week, you can add another one.

Keep a record of your aims and your progress and take pride in every step, knowing that you're on your way to enjoying the miracle of sight for life.

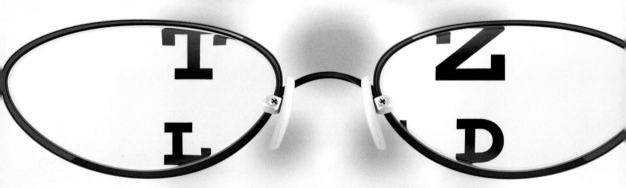

How good is your eyesight?

3

Even if you were fortunate enough to have had near-perfect eyesight when you were young, you will have noticed some changes in your late thirties or early forties. This chapter explains in detail how to assess your sight (the second stage of the plan) and find out just how good it is now, how to improve it, if necessary, and how to deal with any difficulties you already have.

You will learn about some of the common sight problems that may mean you need glasses or contact lenses. While even a minor deterioration in your eyesight can be alarming, as well as inconvenient and irritating, it is reassuring to know that this is rarely due to a serious eye disorder –

though you should always seek professional advice to make sure. Most common difficulties are easy to deal with and there is no need for them to affect your enjoyment of life – or your health.

EVERY OTHER YEAR

You should have a routine eye test every two years – or more often if your doctor or optician recommends it. If you haven't had a test in the past two years, arrange one as soon as possible – you'll normally need to contact an optician and make an appointment. This is especially important if you have recently experienced any sight problems. While the normal changes that occur as we get older are the most likely cause, there is always a risk that something more serious has gone wrong. Some conditions require medical help, described in chapter 4. This chapter explains what a standard eye test can show, and what can be done about any problems that are detected.

WHY EYE TESTS MATTER

It's important to have regular eye tests because potentially serious conditions, such as glaucoma (if left untreated) or cataracts, are silent enemies – they are not usually painful, they appear gradually and do not necessarily produce any symptoms. In the early stages, their effect on vision may be minimal and deterioration too slow to notice. Yet, by the time you become aware of a change, it may be too late. Glaucoma, for instance, is perfectly treatable if caught early, but can cause blindness if ignored.

It's also worth noting that regular eye tests can reveal other problems, such as diabetes and high blood pressure, so you can catch them early, too, before they damage your general health. And every driver should have his or her sight tested regularly to avoid endangering themselves and others.

CAN I GET A FREE TEST?

Many of us are entitled to free eye tests on the NHS, and sometimes also to a voucher that will cover part of the cost of any glasses or contact lenses needed. If you are in any of the following categories, you don't have to pay:

- Aged over 60.
- Aged under 16, or under 19 and in full-time education.
- Receiving certain benefits.
- Requiring complex or powerful lenses.
- Registered blind or partially sighted.
- Already diagnosed with or at risk of glaucoma.
- Over 40 with a close relative (mother, father, brother or sister) who has or had glaucoma.
- Diagnosed with diabetes.
- A regular computer user in paid employment (your employer must by law pay for a test).

Home testing If you cannot visit an optician, you can still have an NHS eye test. Ask your local Primary Care Trust (PCT) for a list of domiciliary eye examination providers who will conduct home tests. Call NHS Direct on 0845 4647 for the contact details for the PCT that covers your area.

10 normal age-related eye changes

You may have noticed some slight changes in your vision. Look at the list of questions below. Is 'yes' your answer to one or more of them? If so, your eyes are probably undergoing the predictable changes that often start when we are in our late thirties or early forties. But there is no need to worry as this is perfectly natural and there is much that you can do.

☐ Do you find that it is getting harder to focus close up, especially for activities such as reading small print – newspapers, for example – or threading a needle and sewing?

☐ Do you find yourself holding the newspaper increasingly further away from your eyes?

☐ Do you need more light to see comfortably, especially for close work?

☐ Does it take your eyes longer to adapt to sudden changes in light levels?

☐ Are you finding it harder to see after dark?

☐ Is it getting harder to drive at night?

☐ Are you increasingly dazzled by bright lights – oncoming headlights, for example?

☐ Do your eyes feel sore or irritated, especially after prolonged close work or computer use?

☐ Do you get a sensation of grittiness in your eyes?

☐ Do colours seem somehow less vivid than they once were?

The more 'yes' answers you give, the more likely it is that you are experiencing normal age-related eye changes, and you would be wise to make an appointment to see your optician. Your GP may be able to help with 'gritty' eyes, and there is plenty of practical advice in chapter 5 (pages 105-108) for tackling the problems of night vision.

your eye test

WHAT HAPPENS?

A routine eye test is painless and usually takes less than half an hour. If you already wear glasses or lenses, take them with you. The optician will ask you general questions about your eyes, your health and any medications you are taking. You may be asked about your family history, in case you are at risk of inherited eye conditions, and about your job and hobbies, as these can affect your visual needs and the likelihood of eyestrain or injuries.

The eye test is designed to assess the general state of your eyes and to make sure that they work together in a coordinated way and that the eye muscles are properly balanced. It can also indicate other health problems – high blood pressure or raised cholesterol, for example – that aren't directly related to your eyes. The optician will test your eyesight for both distant and near vision, and establish the correct strength of any lenses you may need. At the end of the eye test you will be given either a prescription for glasses or contact lenses, or a statement to confirm that your eyesight is fine without correction.

THE OPTICIAN'S TORCH

An instrument called an ophthalmoscope is used to examine the eye. It is like a long thin torch, with a bright light that the optician shines through the pupil, and a magnifying lens through which he or she can examine the back of the eye. An ophthalmoscope is used for the following tests:

- **Pupil reflexes** Normal pupils constrict or narrow under bright light; the light from the ophthalmoscope will trigger both the direct pupil reflex – narrowing on the same side as the light – and the consensual reflex, in which shining a light in one eye causes the pupil in the other eye to constrict as well. Slow, uneven or abnormal pupil responses can indicate a problem with the nerve supply to the eyes.

- **Red reflexes** The red reflex makes use of the effect that causes 'red eye' in photographs (see page 25). When the optician looks directly at the pupil through the ophthalmoscope from about 30 to 45cm (12 to 18in) away, the light hits the back of the eye and is reflected back in the same line. Normally it looks red, owing to the colour of blood vessels in the retina. If this doesn't happen, then a problem with the cornea, lens or retina might be interfering with the light bouncing back. In this case, you might be referred to an ophthalmologist.

A retina review Your optician will peer into each eye from close range to check that your lens looks healthy and to examine your retina. This involves moving the opthalmoscope around to get a good view of all areas; you may hear a series of clicks as the focus is adjusted. The optician is assessing the state of retinal blood vessels, the optic disc (where the optic nerve joins the eye) and the macula (the area in the centre of the retina responsible for detailed central vision). Because such a strong light is used, you may see 'after images' for a few moments, but these disappear quite quickly.

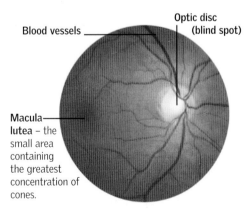

Blood vessels

Optic disc (blind spot)

Macula lutea – the small area containing the greatest concentration of cones.

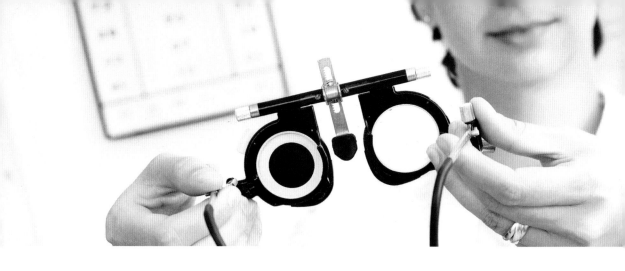

who's who in eye care

Optician is the general name for a professional who supplies visual correction aids, such as glasses or contact lenses, but there are other names for specific eye specialists. What distinguishes an optometrist from an opthalmologist, or an ophthalmic optician from a dispensing optician? Where do ophthalmic medical practitioners and orthoptists fit in? Here is a guide to eye specialists and what they do.

An **optometrist**, previously known as an ophthalmic optician, provides primary eye-care services, performing comprehensive eye tests and also dealing with overall eye health. He or she can examine and test for all eye problems, sight defects and health conditions linked with the eye. Optometrists advise on visual correction, prescribe glasses and contact lenses, give healthcare advice, assess and monitor vision defects and eye disorders, and will refer you to other healthcare providers such as your GP or an ophthalmologist if necessary.

A **dispensing optician** can fill a prescription for glasses given by an optometrist, taking the measurements necessary to ensure that glasses fit properly and advising on style and shape of frames, types of lens and coatings. With special training, a dispensing optician can also fit contact lenses.

An **ophthalmic medical practitioner** is a qualified doctor specialising in eye care and having the same range of functions as an optometrist: examining eyes and diagnosing eye diseases, testing vision, and prescribing glasses or contact lenses.

An **ophthalmologist** is also a qualified doctor who specialises in eye disease and treatment, including performing eye surgery when necessary – so ophthalmologists are also sometimes called ophthalmic surgeons. They usually work in hospitals. There is no need to be anxious if you are referred to an eye doctor – it does not necessarily mean that you will require an operation.

An **orthoptist** is a specialist in the treatment of problems of eye alignment, eye muscle disorders and binocular vision. Orthoptists usually work in a hospital or clinic in close collaboration with ophthalmologists. They assess conditions such as squints and double vision before and after treatment.

Your GP can advise you on eye symptoms and injuries, and refer you for more specialist help if necessary.

WHAT CAN THE OPHTHALMOSCOPE REVEAL?

The optician uses an opthalmoscope to make sure that you do not have eye conditions such as macular degeneration, retinal tears or detachments, as well as to monitor changes that could indicate other conditions, such as diabetes or high cholesterol. If such changes are detected, you are likely to be referred to an eye specialist or to your GP. If a referral is made, your eye examination will have been crucial in detecting a problem sooner rather than later, allowing prompt action to improve your health – or even to save your sight.

GLAUCOMA TESTING

If you are over 40 years old, your eye examination will probably include a check for glaucoma, the tests and treatment for which are explained fully in the next chapter (see pages 88–91). Sometimes glaucoma produces changes in the retina that can be seen through the ophthalmoscope.

You will also be given a 'tonometry' test to measure the pressure inside each of your eyeballs, since high pressure is frequently the cause of glaucoma. For this, you will be asked to look through an eyepiece while a special instrument directs a short puff of air onto the front of each eye in turn – it doesn't hurt but it will make you blink. This is a basic screening test and the results are not conclusive, so your optician may recommend more elaborate tests.

SHARP-EYED

The next part of the eye examination is concerned with sharpness of vision – known as visual acuity (VA). The form you are given after your eye test might include a measure of VA, but this will not necessarily be included in your prescription for glasses or contact lenses.

The aim of this part of the eye test is to find out how well your cones can distinguish fine detail. The optician tests each eye separately, while shielding the other one, and checks your vision with and without correcting lenses. The normal test for this is the familiar chart – called the Snellen chart – which shows rows of letters decreasing in size (see page 56). Your eyesight is graded according to the smallest letters you can read from a fixed distance.

Different charts are used for very young children or for people who cannot recognise letters. One has simple pictures instead of letters; another, the Tumbling E, shows a series of capital Es, facing in different directions. The person being tested has simply to indicate the direction in which the letter is facing.

Continued on p56 ▶

colour spectrum

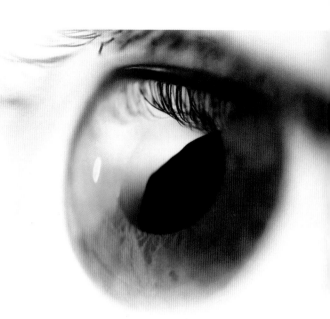

If you have a problem distinguishing colours or an eye condition that impairs colour perception, your optician may check your colour vision as part of your eye test. You must also have the check if you are planning to do a job that requires good colour vision.

The most common test is a series of pictures of coloured dots in which numbers or shapes are picked out in different colours. People with different forms of colour blindness may be unable to distinguish these from the background pattern.

LITTLE BOY PINK ...

Colour blindness occurs when some of the cones – the light-sensitive cells in your retina that detect colour and are responsible for daylight vision – are either missing or not working properly. It is much more common in boys than girls, affecting between 8 and 12 per cent of boys but less than 1 per cent of girls. Colour blindness is usually inherited, so most affected people are born with it – though it is frequently not picked up until someone notices, say, that a child persistently colours the sea pink or confuses the purple crayon with the blue one.

About 99 per cent of all of those people affected have a form of red–green colour blindness. Its severity varies – many colour-blind people are able see some shades of red and green, though they may have difficulty distinguishing between them.

SENSEalert !

COLOUR CONFUSION

If you start to find it difficult to distinguish colours that you used to be able to tell apart, have a check-up. Some diseases, medications, industrial or agricultural chemicals and eye injuries can trigger colour blindness, which may improve through treatment of the disease or by stopping exposure to the drugs or chemicals responsible.

Can you tell red from green?

Try the test below to discover if you are red–green colour-blind. You can also try an online colour vision test at www.city.ac.uk/avrc/colourtest.html, devised by scientists at City University, London. These tests are interesting, but if you are worried about your colour vision, see an optician. Although there is no cure for colour blindness, it is important to have a clear diagnosis.

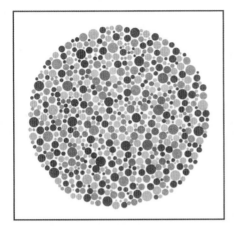

The colour challenge People with normal vision, who look at this standard test will see dots in shades of green forming the number 74, against a background of reddish dots. People who can distinguish some colours but can't see red and green will see the figure 21.

PRACTICALITIES

Being colour-blind does not increase your risk of other eye conditions but it sometimes poses practical frustrations. It may be difficult to distinguish red from green apples or to tell the difference between, say, tomato ketchup and chocolate sauce. More seriously, it can be hard to tell when meat is cooked properly. Matching socks or other clothes, reading maps, home decorating and harvesting strawberries can also cause problems. Some colour-blind people find it difficult to see computer screens clearly. There are some useful tips in chapter 5 about dealing with these everyday hiccups.

Colour blindness won't prevent you from driving. Red and amber traffic lights may look similar, and green may appear dirty white, but the position of the lights will signal their meaning quite clearly – though you may not be able to tell which is lit until you are quite close.

Although there is no cure, colour filters and tinted contact lenses can improve colour differentiation and contrast for some people.

cuttingEDGE

GENE THERAPY FOR COLOUR BLINDNESS?

One day it may be possible to treat hereditary colour blindness by replacing the genes that code for defective or missing cone cells. In animal experiments, Professor Jay Neitz and colleagues at the Medical College of Wisconsin in Milwaukee have successfully injected normal genes directly into the retinas of rats. The human cone gene somehow integrates into the rat retinal cells but, as rats have little colour vision, the full effect is still unknown. Trials in people are still a long way off, but Professor Neitz is convinced that, ultimately, 'gene therapy will cure colour blindness'.

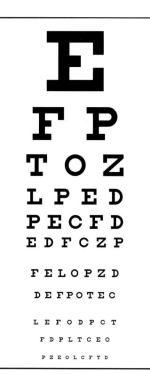

The Snellen chart: can you read the eighth line down from 6m (20ft) away?

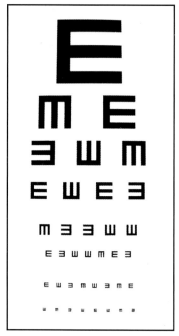

The Tumbling E chart: which direction is each of the letter Es facing?

HOW EYE SIGHT IS MEASURED – THREE DIFFERENT SCALES

Snellen	Metric	Decimal	
20/200	6/60	0.1	(represents legal blindness)
20/100	6/30	0.2	
20/50	6/15	0.4	
20/40	6/12	0.5	
20/30	6/9	0.66	
20/25	6/7.5	0.8	
20/20	6/6	1.0	(normal vision)
20/15	6/4.5	1.33	
20/10	6/3	2.0	(extremely good vision)

WHAT IS 'NORMAL' VISION?

Normal visual acuity is described as 20/20 (or 6/6 in the metric system). It means that you are able to read letters of a particular size – usually the eighth line down on the Snellen chart – at a distance of 20ft (6m). The result is shown as a fraction, and the higher the second number, the worse the vision. So if your result was 20/40 (or 6/12), it would mean that you would need letters twice as large as someone with normal vision in order to see them – or you'd need to be half the distance from the chart.

Your optician may record your test results not as a Snellen fraction but as its corresponding number: 20/20 or 6/6 equals 1.0, while 20/40 or 6/12 equals 0.5 – so, when recorded as a decimal, the higher the number the better your vision. The chart above shows the Snellen and metric fractions and their decimal equivalents.

AVERAGE IS BETTER THAN NORMAL!

Visual acuity tends to improve up to the age of 25, and most young adults with healthy eyes can read the lines of smaller letters under the 20/20 row. This 'better-than-normal' vision will score in the ranges indicated on the Snellen/Metric/Decimal chart, above. In fact the average score for healthy eyes is usually between 20/16 and 20/12, which means average vision is actually better than 20/20 or 'normal'. If your test result is 20/10 (or 6/3 or 2.0), it means that you can see letters 6m (20ft) away that someone with 'normal' eyesight could read from only 3m (10ft).

WHAT YOUR RESULTS MEAN

If you can't read the 20/20 line on the Snellen chart from the required distance, you have what's called 'impaired visual acuity'. You may be shortsighted, longsighted or have astigmatism, or you may have an eye disease such as cataract or macular degeneration. If your acuity is only slightly reduced, to around 20/30 (6/9), you can still drive safely; most European countries, using the metric system, require 6/12 vision or better for a driving licence. If your test results show a Snellen level of 20/60 (6/18) or poorer, you are classified as having impaired vision and probably find it hard to watch television across the room, read signs or recognise friends in the street.

Vision testing with a Snellen chart is not the ultimate arbiter of eyesight. It can measure your ability to distinguish letters at a high contrast to their background from a set distance away in good light but it doesn't necessarily indicate how well you see in real life – from a cat in the road ahead of your car to the kerb on a badly lit street at night.

WHY 20/20 VISION?

Hermann Snellen, the Dutch ophthalmologist who in 1862 devised the chart bearing his name, used the ability to read a particular row of letters simply as a reference point to define standard vision – though it is actually the lower end of the 'normal' range.

It became common practice to view the chart from a distance of 6m (20ft), because this is close to optical infinity – meaning that when you stare at a far-off horizon the light rays reaching your eye are virtually parallel. In consequence, there is very little distortion when the lens in your eye changes shape to focus on larger or smaller letters on the chart.

In English-speaking countries, 20/20 became synonymous with good sight and is also the typical length of eye-examination rooms in the USA. If the room is smaller, the chart can be read in a mirror. In Britain, many opticians have the chart itself placed behind the chair where you sit, and you are asked to read the letters in a mirror on the wall in front of you.

NEAR VISION

Your optician will also test how well you focus on things close up, using a hand-held card with small chunks of text in progressively smaller print. You will be asked to hold the card at a set distance, usually about 40cm (15in) from your eyes. Your optician will record the smallest text that you can read, and the distance at which you can do so. The letter sizes on the card are calculated to show the equivalent of 20/20 vision and variations either side (20/10, 20/40 and so on), with and without glasses or lenses.

Most young people who score well for distant vision will also score 20/20 or better for near vision. But when we reach our forties, many of us notice that we need to hold the print further and further away in order to read it. This is known as presbyopia, and is nothing to worry about (see page 67). All it means is that we need reading glasses.

eye tests **online**

If you have access to the internet, you may have come across various web-based eye tests and questionnaires that you can print out and complete, or try out while sitting at your computer. Contrary to what you might expect, experts now suggest that these tests can be useful. Specialist ophthalmology journals increasingly report that internet eye testing can achieve comparable results to conventional testing, although the difficulties of taking the tests under standard conditions (such as clarity, distance and brightness) can make the results unreliable.

Why not have a go at some of them (the web addresses are listed below)? But don't forget that these are no substitute for a professional eye test – use them as a back-up between your regular eye tests, not instead of them, and always seek professional advice if you develop any new eye or vision symptoms.

Online tests
For distant vision: www.eyes-and-vision.com/take-the-snellen-eye-test-online.html
For colour vision: http://colorvisiontesting.com/online%20test.htm
For macular degeneration: http://www.eyesight.org/Eye_Test/eye_test.html

Questionnaires
To find out if you need a professional eye test: http://doineedaneyetest.com/
To assess age-related changes: http://www.agingeye.net/onlinetest.php

getting **back** into focus

If you need glasses or lenses, your optician will use a special pair of testing frames – much bulkier than normal glasses – into which he or she can slot different lenses. You will be asked to look at various charts and symbols to see what works best. The optician will choose the best lens for each eye and write you a prescription. You can have the prescription made up by the same optician or take it elsewhere – glasses and lenses are expensive, so people often shop around for the best deal.

WHY WE NEED GLASSES
Did you know that almost 70 per cent of people in Britain wear either glasses or contact lenses? So, if you have been told you need a visual aid, you are firmly in the majority. Your prescription aims to correct whatever type of refractive error you have.

All refractive errors involve a problem with the way that light rays entering the eye are bent inwards to reach a focal point (the place where the image is clearest). As explained in chapter 1, if the focal point is not on the retina, the eye is unable to form a clear image (see page 22).

When you look at something close up, light needs to be bent more than if you are looking into the distance. Most of this bending is done by the cornea, which provides about 70 per cent of the focusing power of the eye – the lens simply fine-tunes the image. In an eye with normal vision, the curvature of the cornea is exactly matched with the length of the eyeball. This means that it can bend light coming from near or far and, after additional focusing by the lens, bring it to a focal point precisely on the retina, allowing crisp vision whatever the distance.

shortsightedness

If you are shortsighted – the most common sight problem, and the most likely defect when you're young – either your eyeball is too long or your cornea is too steep, so light rays coming from a distance are bent too much. The focal point forms in front of the retina, and by the time the rays reach the retina they have spread apart again, so the image is no longer in focus. To someone who is shortsighted, distant objects look blurred,

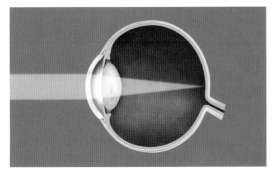

The focal point in a normal eye

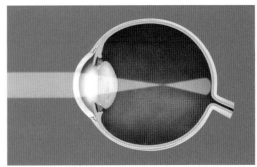

The focal point in a shortsighted eye

though those close up are seen clearly. If you have been told that you have short sight (also called near sight or myopia), you probably discovered that you needed glasses during your childhood or in your teens.

SPOTTED BY THE TEACHER

Most babies are born with a degree of longsightedness, so short sight is rare before the age of five. It tends to start in late childhood, roughly between the ages of 8 and 12, but is frequently not picked up until adolescence. That is because shortsightedness develops so gradually that children don't notice that fuzzy vision is a problem or realise that their sight is any different from other people's. As a consequence, myopia is easily overlooked unless a child undergoes regular eye tests.

It is not uncommon for short sight to be picked up for the first time when a teacher notices that a child has difficulty seeing the blackboard (or, these days, the interactive whiteboard) although he or she can read perfectly normally close up. Sometimes an alert games teacher may notice that a child has become less coordinated or less good at sports.

Shortsightedness generally develops at any time up to the age of 25, but after that it is much less likely. The chances are that if you're over 30 you have escaped – but read on to discover what causes myopia, and why people in the modern world may still be at risk even when they get older.

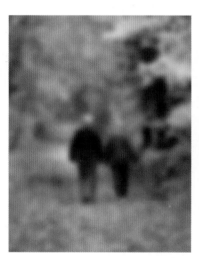 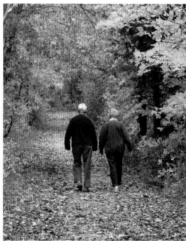

Lifting the fog
People who are shortsighted see distant objects or people as a blur (left) but properly prescribed glasses or contact lenses will correct the problem and provide clear vision (right).

If you are shortsighted, it probably got worse during the early years and stabilised in your late teens or early twenties. Myopia does not usually progress once someone has stopped growing, though the earlier it starts the more severe it is likely to be.

THE EFFECTS OF SHORTSIGHTEDNESS

Shortsightedness makes distant objects look blurred and also causes tired eyes and headaches, but it is not detrimental to your overall eye health. In fact, as you get older, you may have an advantage over your normally sighted friends – your eyes effectively have a built-in reading prescription. You won't necessarily escape presbyopia (see page 67) altogether, but you will probably notice it later and to a lesser extent, so you'll be able to carry on reading without glasses for longer. Most shortsighted people are affected to a mild or medium degree, but about one in 20 has high-degree myopia. This is associated with an increased risk of eye disorders in later life, so if your optician tells you that you have high-degree myopia you should be extra vigilant about reporting eye symptoms as you get older and, of course, making sure that you have regular eye tests.

WHY AM I SHORTSIGHTED?

Shortsightedness is partly hereditary. If one of your parents is shortsighted, you run about a 30 per cent risk of developing myopia, and this increases to 55 per cent if both your parents are shortsighted. The severity of the condition also runs in families, so if you have a very shortsighted parent you are at greater risk of developing severe myopia. The same applies to your children if you or your partner are shortsighted, and to your grandchildren if their parents are affected. What's more, whereas until recently genetic influences were believed to be the main factor in the development of short sight, recently a new risk has emerged – so even if you are not affected, shortsightedness could still affect your children or grandchildren.

non-SENSE X

WEARING GLASSES MAKES SHORTSIGHTEDNESS WORSE

It is a myth that wearing glasses or contact lenses somehow weakens your eyes and makes the problem of short sight worse. Not wearing them when you need to can, however, contribute to eyestrain, and is dangerous when you are driving or operating machinery, for example.

ON THE INCREASE

Recent surveys in Western Europe and the USA suggest that, on average, up to one in four people is shortsighted. But in the last few decades there have been rapid increases in rates of myopia in most countries around the world – and in Asia, the worst-affected region, the problem has been described as an 'epidemic'. Is there something in our environment or our behaviour that might be influencing the trend?

Scientists now think that myopia results from an interplay between genetic and environmental factors. It could be that, during crucial periods of their development, children and adolescents with an inherited likelihood of shortsightedness are even more vulnerable to other influences that promote its development. Although reading and close work have been implicated, a peculiarly modern factor would seem to be young people spending long hours using computers and playing computer games.

Continued on p65 ▶

short sight –
a modern phenomenon

Medical experts are aware that short sight often runs in families but no one has pinpointed why people are developing short sight in such increasing numbers. The evidence is complicated and sometimes conflicting.

Recent studies of twins in Britain and Denmark indicate that inheritance causes or contributes to about 86 per cent of all cases of shortsightedness, which suggests a strong genetic influence. But numerous population studies also show that myopia is especially common among certain groups – such as university students – which could mean that environmental factors are partly responsible; close work, such as reading and writing, is the prime suspect. Another potential culprit is artificial light, while some scientists think that inadequate physical activity and poor diet also play a role.

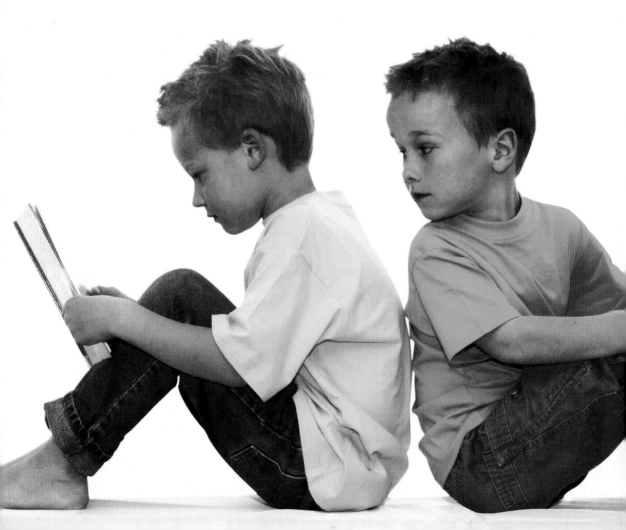

THE LINK WITH CLOSE WORK

Although rates of shortsightedness vary between countries, age trends are similar across the world. Short sight is rare before school age and becomes progressively more common in the school years. In the USA it increases more than sevenfold, from around 2 per cent of six-year-olds to 15 per cent of 15-year-olds. Research has shown that shortsightedness in children progresses faster in the school year than during the summer holidays.

> Short sight is rare before school age and becomes progressively more common in the school years.

And the incidence of shortsightedness peaks among university students – at the time of most intensive close work. For example, it has been reported that virtually all medical students in Taiwan are myopic. In Singapore, the situation is particularly worrying. According to the Singapore National Eye Centre, myopia appears early, high-degree myopia is common, and the number affected has vastly increased in three generations.

Today, myopia affects 25 per cent of seven-year-olds, 33 per cent of nine-year-olds, 50 per cent of 12-year-olds and over 80 per cent of 18-year-old males in Singapore. Thirty years ago, just 25 per cent of male army recruits were shortsighted. Although people of Chinese extraction run a high genetic risk of shortsightedness, the rates in Singapore are much higher even than those of nearby Taiwan and Hong Kong. Scientists think that this points to environmental as well as genetic influences – specifically highlighting the huge emphasis on reading and other close work in the rigorous Singaporean education system.

NURTURE VS. NATURE

Classic studies of Alaskan Inuit children showed a dramatic increase in myopia following the introduction of a 'westernised' lifestyle and, especially, of compulsory education. In an investigation into Alaskan Inuit families, first reported in the *American Journal of Optometry and Archives of American Academy of Optometry* in 1969, only two out of 130 parents (who had all lived a traditional life of hunting and fishing) were myopic but more than 60 per cent of their children had measurable short sight. Dr Francis Young, who led the research team, concluded that long periods of reading at school were to blame.

ADULT RISK?

Shortsightedness also seems to be developing in adults not previously thought at risk. A major US investigation, the Framingham Offspring Eye Study, showed a marked increase in myopia among younger adults. Scientists think that emphasis on prolonged close work, in education and in business life, means that our eyes are continually accommodating to focus on computer screens, reading or writing material. They get less chance to relax compared with the eyes of people who spend most of their days out of doors, and this may cause eye changes that lead to short sight.

NIGHT LIGHTS AND SHORTSIGHTEDNESS

One study at the University of Pennsylvania Medical Center and the Children's Hospital of Philadelphia reported that the prevalence of myopia among children aged two to 16 increased from 10 per cent in those who, as babies, had slept in complete darkness to 34 per cent in those who had slept with a night light – and a staggering 55 per cent among those whose parents had left on a full room light.

PREVENTION

Not everyone agrees on what's causing the short-sight 'epidemic', but it's wise to follow the tips in chapter 2 for reducing eyestrain when doing close work. And many experts believe that prolonged computer use exacerbates the trend, so protect your sight by following the advice on how best to set up a computer workstation (see pages 36-37) and by taking frequent breaks.

THE LINK WITH ARTIFICIAL LIGHT

Not only do we spend far more time than previous generations on close work, but we also spend much of this time working under artificial light. Several studies in recent years have led scientists to suspect that this might explain the rising rates of myopia in urban societies. Perhaps your mother was right to warn you not to read by torchlight under the bedclothes. But why should artificial light be harmful? In 2007, in the journal *Medical Hypotheses*, California eye specialist Dr S.B. Prepas speculated that close focusing in the absence of ultraviolet light – which is present in natural sunlight but not artificial light – could provoke eye changes that lead to short sight. Other studies in children and university students suggest that the development of shortsightedness may also be accelerated by 'darkness deprivation' – the failure to rest your eyes properly caused by sleeping in half-lit rooms. (See 'What's the evidence?', above)

So, if you do a lot of reading, studying or computer work, it may be better for your eyes to do it during the day – ideally at a desk near a window – rather than in the evenings. At night, turn off the light and enjoy a long sleep in a completely dark room.

FOOD AND FITNESS

As we said in the last chapter, obesity and diabetes have both been linked to modern diets high in starches, which may also contribute to short sight. In fact, some scientists believe that dietary changes offer a more convincing explanation than close work for the myopia epidemic. Also, shortsighted children spend significantly less time playing sports, and so less time outdoors, than their normally sighted peers. This could be because of their short sight; on the other hand, their short sight could be due to more time spent reading or a lack of daylight. Better light levels outdoors make near-vision focusing easier, while reduced sun exposure may contribute to the development of short sight. Or sports activities could, perhaps, have a truly protective effect on the eyes – consistent with suggestions that physical exercise boosts eye health.

long**sightedness**

People who have long sight (also called far sightedness, hypermetropia or hyperopia) can see distant objects quite clearly but have difficulty focusing on things close up – the opposite problem to those with short sight. Longsighted vision occurs because the eyeball is too short or the cornea is not sufficiently curved, so light rays from nearby objects are still too far apart by the time they reach the retina. As demonstrated by the diagram on page 66, the focal point is effectively behind the retina, making nearby objects look blurred, while things in the distance are in sharp focus.

Like myopia, longsightedness also runs in families and seems to be mostly inherited. Most babies are born with a degree of longsightedness, but children's flexible lenses can compensate for this, so fewer than one in ten are still longsighted between the ages of 5 and 20.

SENSEalert

LONGSIGHTED CHILDREN

In children, whose vision is still developing, being longsighted can lead to other problems, such as double vision, squint (where the eyes are not properly aligned) and 'lazy eye' or amblyopia (where normal visual development is impaired because one eye doesn't work properly). This again underlines the importance of regular eye tests since these conditions could result in permanent damage to a child's sight.

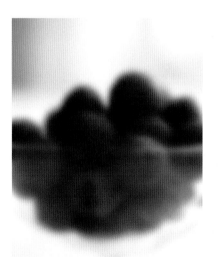

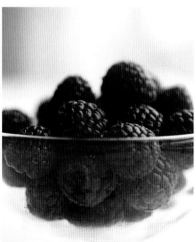

What am I eating?

Longsightedness, which is mostly inherited, makes near objects seem blurred (left) but, like short sight, can be readily corrected (right) by using appropriately prescribed glasses or contact lenses.

WHEN LONG SIGHT RETURNS

Whereas generally your risk of developing short sight diminishes as you get older, the incidence of longsightedness increases with age, affecting one in six adults aged 40 to 45, half of those over 65, and as many as two-thirds of people over 80. Ageing doesn't actually cause long sight, but any

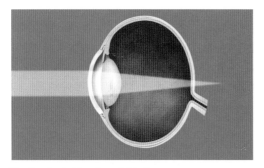
The focal point in a longsighted eye

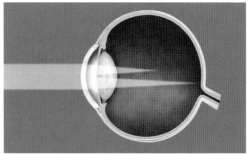
Multiple focal points in an astigmatic eye

inherent longsightedness becomes more apparent with age because your lens gets stiffer, so its ability to compensate – as it did when you were younger – is reduced, making it more difficult to focus on close-up objects. As this process occurs gradually, you may not even realise that you have a vision problem. You might be aware instead that your eyes feel tired or sore and you might get headaches after prolonged close work.

Longsighted people are at greater risk of developing glaucoma (see page 88), so should be especially careful to have regular eye tests. There are few other complications for adults, although most longsighted people need progressively stronger glasses or lenses.

astigmatism

Astigmatism means that the shape of the eyeball is distorted, and is longer in one direction than another, rather like a rugby ball. This means that either the cornea or, less often, the lens, is not smoothly curved like the surface of a ping-pong ball, as it should be. The irregular curvature means that light entering the eye is bent more in one direction than another. Light rays do not come to a focus at a single point but produce two or more focal points, so only part of an image is in focus at any time. This makes images appear blurred or wavy.

Astigmatism can occur with long or short sight, and most people have it to some degree. If it's mild, it does not need treatment. If you are experiencing blurring for near and distant vision, or any other symptoms – such as squinting, eyestrain or fatigue when doing close work – you need to get your eyes tested. If you are found to have astigmatism and you do a lot of driving or spend long hours in front of a computer, you will probably need some form of correcting lenses. The condition can be hereditary and is frequently present from birth. Like longsightedness, it tends to get worse with age. It can also develop with some eye diseases or following injury or surgery; it could even be caused by habitually adopting an asymmetric posture or reading at an angle. Sometimes, a cyst on the eyelid causes astigmatism; in this case, once the cyst clears up then so does the astigmatism.

Presbyopia – perfectly natural

If you are in your forties, you may find that you can now legitimately wear funky glasses to hide those laughter lines. Whether you are shortsighted, longsighted or have had perfect vision for most of your life, there are age-related eye changes that few people – if anyone – can avoid.

By the time we reach 60, most of us will need reading glasses for a condition called presbyopia that makes our near vision less good than it once was. Scientists think that presbyopia is caused by a combination of thicker, harder, less flexible lenses and less efficient, more lax eye muscles – which makes it harder for our eyes to focus on objects close up. Eventually the near point – the closest distance from which the eye can create a sharp image on the retina – is farther away from the eye than the reading distance.

By the time we reach 60, most of us will need reading glasses for a condition called presbyopia that makes our near vision less good than it once was.

If you find that you are having to hold books, newspapers and menus at arm's length in order to read what seems like increasingly hazy print, you have probably got presbyopia. It is virtually inevitable and usually becomes more noticeable between the ages of 40 and 50. It is worse in poor light and improves in sunlight, because pupil narrowing improves focus. Prolonged close work may cause headaches or eyestrain. Presbyopia will run its course irrespective of whether you wear glasses; glasses will compensate for the problem rather than contributing to it.

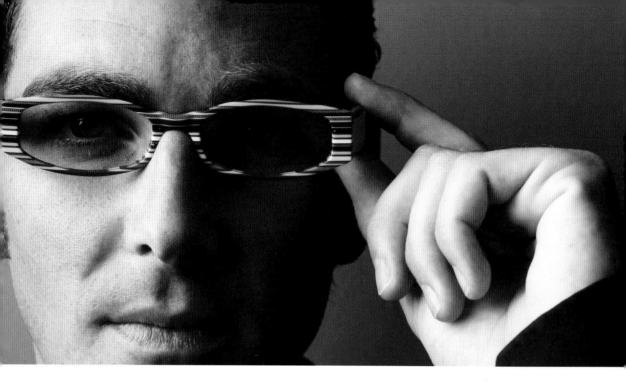

looking good – today's fashion accessories

If you need glasses, take heart. 'Eyewear' has come a long way since the days of ugly utilitarian frames and bottle-glass lenses. 'Glasses' are so-called because originally the lenses were made of glass; nowadays they are usually made of a special lightweight plastic. The curvature and thickness of the lens (and therefore the weight) depends on the degree of visual correction required, but the combination of modern lens manufacturing technology and a wide choice of lightweight frames means that today's spectacles can be an attractive fashion accessory.

LIGHTWEIGHT LENSES FOR ALL

New 'high-index' materials, with extra light-bending capacity, have made possible the manufacture of high-powered lenses that are thinner, lighter and less distorting when viewed from the front, so that they look good even if you are extremely shortsighted (and would once have needed the dreaded thick lenses). Aspheric lenses, in which the curvature changes gradually, bulge less and provide better vision with less distortion at the edges. They are suitable for correcting both long and short sight.
If your prescription includes a correction for astigmatism, the lenses will be specially ground so that they bend light more in one direction than

another, to neutralise the irregular curvature of your cornea. These are called toric lenses. You can have your lenses coated with a variety of finishes:

- Anti-reflection coatings can be useful for computer work or night driving; they can also make thicker lenses look thinner, again improving their appearance.
- Scratch-resistant coatings help to protect against damage and are especially useful for children and sports players.
- A scratch-resistant coating can be combined with a coating that is specially designed to protect your eyes against ultraviolet (UV) rays in sunlight – though some lens materials have inherent anti-UV protection.

LENS TYPES

Before you consider your choice of frame and lens coating, you need to know what type of glasses you require.

Single-vision Single-vision spectacles are the simplest type of glasses in that they correct for shortsightedness or longsightedness with a single prescription. Manufactured lenses in glasses (and contact lenses) work in exactly the same way as the lens in your eye: they bend light rays.

If you are longsighted, a convex lens – which is thicker in the centre than at the edges just like the lens in your eye – adds to the focusing power of your own eye to pull the focal point forwards onto the retina, so that near images appear sharp again.

If you are shortsighted, your lens will be concave – thinner in the centre than at the edge. This bends light rays outwards, compensating for the excess bending produced by your eyes and pushing the focal point back towards the retina, so that distant objects come back into focus.

Reading glasses If you have presbyopia, a pair of glasses just for reading may be the answer. Even if you also require a prescription for distant vision, you could have a separate pair of reading glasses to wear when you need to do close work. If you usually wear contact lenses (see pages 70–74) for distant vision, your optician can prescribe reading glasses that will work while you are wearing your lenses. You can buy simple magnifying reading glasses over the counter without a prescription. Presbyopia tends to worsen with time, though, so you may need to wear increasingly strong reading glasses as you get older.

Bifocals Bifocals enable two different prescriptions to be combined in a single lens, for people who need one correction for regular wear and another for close work. The upper part of the lens corrects distant vision and the lower part close vision, with a distinct dividing line between the two halves. There are also trifocals, which have three sections for distant, intermediate and near vision. However, bifocals and trifocals do not suit everyone and the sudden jump from one correction to another can be irksome, so varifocals are now more often prescribed.

Varifocals These operate similarly to bifocals for people who need more than one correction but, as the name implies, use a graduated correction in which the power of the lens changes smoothly from one prescription to the other without visible divisions. They make possible clear vision at all distances, though it can take a while to get used to them.

invisible assets

Contact lenses provide a virtually weightless and invisible alternative to glasses and give an unobstructed view across the whole visual field. They correct vision in exactly the same way as glasses, and the technology has advanced by leaps and bounds since the days of rigid, daily-wear lenses that took weeks to get accustomed to and also required a medicine chest full of cleaning, disinfecting and storage products. Modern lenses are so comfortable that you can forget you're wearing them within seconds of insertion. They are available in soft, disposable, gas-permeable, extended-wear and even tinted varieties. In the past, you may have been told that lenses were not suitable for you; today, that is probably no longer true.

If you have presbyopia, you may now be able to wear either bifocal or varifocal contact lenses. And lenses can

SENSE-sational

MONOVISION: THE BEST OF BOTH WORLDS?

A new way to deal with combined presbyopia and myopia is to correct one eye for near vision and the other for distant vision, a technique called 'monovision'. This can be achieved either with contact lenses or by laser surgery (see page 75). It is a compromise, however, and not suitable if you need really sharp distance vision for, say, playing golf, or if you do a lot of close work. The brain must get used to each eye 'dominating' at a different distance – at first, it might even make you feel giddy or sick. But many people adapt fast and it's a way to avoid multiple prescriptions.

Modern lenses are so comfortable that you can forget you're wearing them within seconds.

now be made to counteract astigmatism, although if your cornea is too uneven, you may have to wear hard lenses rather than soft ones, which would simply mould to the irregular shape.

HARD OR SOFT?

The contact lenses available today are made of a variety of materials, and length-of-wear times and disposal periods also vary. Your optician can advise which are best for you.

Rigid Now rarely prescribed, rigid lenses can be difficult to get used to. They deprive the cornea of oxygen and can be worn only during the day. They are sometimes recommended for people with severe astigmatism.

Gas permeable These lenses are made of a material that allows oxygen to pass through them but, being hard, they also take time to get accustomed to. Less widely used than soft lenses, they may be recommended for people with severe astigmatism or presbyopia.

Soft The original soft contact lenses are made from a squashy material combining water and plastic, called a hydrogel, which is not gas permeable but allows oxygen to reach the eye through its water content. Newer variants combine water with silicone, making them gas permeable, so they can be worn even when you are sleeping. You can also get versions that alter the colour of your eyes. A soft lens is slightly larger than the eye's iris, so it can be seen if someone looks closely.

Hybrid Some lenses have a soft outer rim combined with a rigid, gas-permeable centre, providing comfort in addition to the slightly superior visual qualities of a hard lens.

cuttingEDGE

LENSES THAT ALSO DELIVER MEDICATION

Medicinal eye drops are difficult and messy to administer. When you do succeed in getting them into your eye, they mix with tears and end up running down your face – wasting about 95 per cent of the medication, according to experts. Even the drops that stay in the eye provide a high drug concentration for only about 2 minutes before they are diluted; meanwhile, some of the fluid may drain into the nose, from where the drug can get into the bloodstream, possibly causing unwanted side-effects.

Researchers at the University of Florida have now developed a soft contact lens material that binds to and slowly releases medicinal drugs directly into the eye. These lenses could be worn for up to two weeks, all the time delivering the correct dose direct to the eyes. If successful in clinical trials, they could one day replace eye drops. And lenses could also incorporate antibiotics, to reduce the high risk of bacterial infections that lens wearers normally face.

Daily wear Hard and gas-permeable lenses must be removed and cleaned every night; you can't sleep in them. On the plus side, they last for about a year before you need to replace them. You can also get daytime-wear soft lenses that last from three to 12 months and soft 'disposable' lenses designed for daytime wear for shorter periods before planned replacement.

Extended wear Sometimes called 'continuous wear' lenses, these are soft lenses that you can sleep in. Depending on the type, you can keep them in for between a week and a month. Then they must be replaced. They are more expensive than daytime-wear lenses, but you save on cleaning products.

Daily disposable The ultimate in consumer eyewear are soft lenses that you simply throw away at the end of each day. Disposable lenses are the most expensive option if you use them all the time, but users swear by them and feel they are worth every penny.

Even if your lenses incorporate anti-UV protection, you still need good-quality sunglasses when out in the sun.

lens care

Most people adapt quickly and wear their lenses happily and successfully, delighting in the freedom it gives them from carrying and wearing glasses each day. But about one in 20 lens wearers each year will encounter problems. Most of these are minor difficulties, usually caused by wearing lenses for too long, failing to follow simple hygiene rules, sensitivity to lens cleaning solutions or poor lens fit. The biggest danger with lenses is infection, but if you follow the safety guidelines on page 74, your eyes will have a long and happy relationship with their lenses.

When you are prescribed lenses for the first time, you will have frequent check-ups for a while, and usually annual examinations thereafter. Make sure you follow care-and-wear routines to the letter and, if any problems do arise, seek help promptly.

SOLUTION TO SOLUTIONS

Hypersensitivity to contact lens solutions is quite common. Most solutions today are multipurpose; one fluid can be used for cleaning, disinfection and storage. But if your eyes become irritated, sore or red and you have difficulty wearing the lenses, you may be sensitive to the fluid. Change to a different solution or try one that is preservative-free.

GRIT IN THE EYE

Pain, watering, redness and a sensation that feels as if you have dust in your eye, which doesn't go away when you blink, could indicate that you have scratched your cornea with a piece of grit trapped behind a lens. Take out the lens as soon as you notice the symptoms and wash your eye with clean water or, ideally, a sterile saline solution (available from pharmacies). If you keep your eye closed as much as possible and don't rub it, the scratch should heal by itself within a couple of days.

PROTEIN DEPOSITS

Sometimes, you may experience an immune response to irritation when your eyelids rub on protein deposits that have built up on the surface of contact lenses. Symptoms include reduced tolerance to the lenses, itching, blurred vision and a mucous discharge, and will affect between 1 and 3 per cent of all lens wearers at some time. The scientific name – 'giant papillary conjunctivitis' – sounds alarming, but the condition is easily dealt with. See your optician, who will probably advise more vigorous cleaning or replacement of the lenses; you may also be prescribed medication and advised to reduce the amount of time you wear your lenses.

YOU STILL NEED SUNGLASSES

Although contact lens material frequently incorporates protection against ultraviolet rays, the lens doesn't cover the whole of your eye – so you still need good-quality sunglasses when out in the sun.

BE PREPARED

If you depend on your lenses to lead life normally, it is important to have a pair of glasses as back-up in case of emergency.

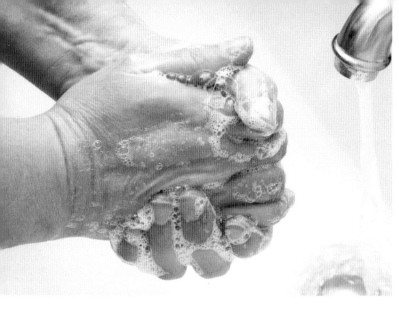

WASH YOUR
HANDS AND
DRY THEM
THOROUGHLY
BEFORE
HANDLING
YOUR LENSES.

safe lens use

Contact lenses are an invaluable visual aid but they need to be respected and looked after carefully, and so do your eyes. You can ensure a lifetime of healthy eyes by following the instructions for daily or weekly lens care for your type of lenses that were given to you by your optician – including how long you can wear them for – and by observing the following guidelines.

- Use only the solutions recommended by your optician. There is a wide choice of 'one-bottle' systems – all-in-ones which are the easiest and quickest to use. But if your eyes are particularly sensitive, a hydrogen peroxide system may be better.
- Never use tap water to rinse your lenses or their cases. There is a risk of microbial and amoebic contamination from tap water, which can cause severe eye infections.
- Don't use saliva to moisten your lenses – it's full of bacteria.
- Take your lenses out before showering or using a sauna, steam room or jacuzzi.
- If possible, don't wear your lenses for swimming or water sports unless you are also wearing goggles with a firm seal. Otherwise the lenses may float from your eyes, or they could absorb the pool water, with the risk of infection or pain from the chlorine.
- Wash your hands and dry them thoroughly before handling your lenses.
- After inserting your lenses, immediately discard the storage solution.
- Air-dry the storage case and fill with fresh solution before storing lenses overnight.
- Replace your storage case every month to stop a build-up of contamination.
- Don't wear your lenses for longer than the recommended time.
- Replace lenses and solutions at the recommended intervals. Replacing lenses prevents discomfort, dryness, blurred vision and allergic reactions that can result from a build-up of protein deposits on the lenses. This is especially true of soft lenses that you wear overnight.
- Never reuse a daily disposable contact lens. Putting in new, sterile lenses every day is the healthiest way to wear contact lenses; reusing them could damage your eyes.
- Put your lenses in before applying make-up, and take them out before taking it off.
- If you develop any symptoms, take out your lenses and don't try wearing them again until you've seen your optician – make an appointment right away.

laser surgery

Many people have undergone laser surgery to correct their vision and achieve complete freedom from glasses and lenses. Originally used mainly for short sight, it can now correct mild long sight and even astigmatism. The procedure takes less than an hour and can be done without a hospital stay, usually in specialised clinics using anaesthetic eye drops. Patients are often back at work within a few days, though you may not be able to drive for a couple of weeks and may need to wear sunglasses for several months as the eyes are more sensitive to light after laser surgery. Both eyes can be corrected in one operation but surgeons usually operate on one eye at a time, waiting a few days or weeks before correcting the other to see how the first eye has responded. If you decide to have laser surgery, you can organise it yourself, without going through your GP, even though it involves specialist treatment. A number of hospital eye departments offer the procedure, but it is not available on the NHS.

Laser surgery is performed only on adults (generally people over 21, to be sure that the eye has developed fully), and on healthy eyes with a stable prescription for visual correction for at least three years. Interestingly, in some occupations laser surgery may be an obstacle to employment. It may cause problems for divers, for example, and the police force used to exclude people who had had the surgery, but the bar has been lifted since the advent of the newer surgical procedures.

thinkSENSE ● ● ●

DO YOUR HOMEWORK

Although laser surgery is usually safe, it makes sense to ensure that it is carried out by a properly trained surgeon in a well-equipped clinic. There are no specific qualifications for doctors performing the surgery, but the Royal College of Ophthalmologists recommends that they should be fully trained ophthalmologists with specialist training in laser use, and that patients should check whether the clinic or hospital where they are considering treatment follows the Royal College guidelines for laser refractive surgery. The college produces a guide to the surgery, available on its website (www.rcophth.ac.uk/about/public/laser-refractive-surgery). Clinics offering laser surgery in the UK must be registered with the Healthcare Commission. All premises are inspected annually, inspection reports appear on their website (www.healthcarecommission.org.uk) or you can call their helpline on 0845 6013012.

THREE TECHNIQUES

The three main types of laser surgery all work by reshaping the cornea. Your surgeon will advise on which is the most suitable for your eyes.

● PRK (Photorefractive keratectomy) This is the original operation and is rarely used nowadays. It is more painful than the other options and

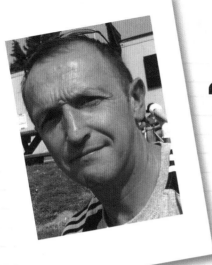

'brilliant' for sport

Roy Brady

'**I** was never comfortable wearing glasses; it always felt awkward,' says Roy Brady, a general builder and handyman, who had laser treatment to correct his shortsightedness 15 years ago.

'When I played squash, I hated it when sweat ran down my face onto my glasses but I couldn't see any distance without them. I tried contact lenses but they were uncomfortable and my eyes often became very dry. That's when I thought about laser surgery.

'Carol, my then partner, had the treatment first. We had checked as much as we could but it wasn't as easy to research as it is now with the internet. So she went to Optimax because they had already done thousands of these operations. Carol's treatment was very successful, so I thought I'd try it myself.

'It was brilliant. I ended up with better-than-perfect vision. There were no drawbacks at all. It was expensive but I've never regretted it.'

'They did one eye at a time. First I had a consultation and an eye test to find out if I was suitable for the treatment. Then I went back for the operation. It only took a couple of minutes. They put eye drops in to anaesthetise the eye, then used a laser to reshape the lens. It was a bit sore for a day or two but after a week the eye was back to normal. Once I knew the first eye operation was successful, I went back – about six months later – and had the second eye corrected.

'And it was brilliant. I ended up with better-than-perfect vision. There were no drawbacks at all. It was expensive at the time but I've never regretted it. It was a total success. I love sports like squash, diving and windsurfing, so for me, it was all about convenience – and vanity,' he adds.

'I also think I was fortunate. Other people have not had the same success – when I had it done, the surgery was not as precise as it is today. It's much more sophisticated and accurate now – and, actually, no more expensive!'

Now in his forties, Roy has, however, noticed some natural deterioration in his near sight. 'I'm beginning to need glasses for reading but my distant vision is as good as ever.'

healing times are longer. It involves scraping away the top layer of the surface of the cornea, then changing its shape with a laser.

- LASEK (Laser epithelial keratomileusis) This method has largely been replaced by LASIK (see below). It uses alcohol to loosen the surface of the cornea, so that it can be lifted out of the way before the laser is used. Afterwards, the surface of the cornea is put back in place. Healing may be slightly painful, and recovery takes up to a week.
- LASIK (Laser Assisted In Situ Keratomileusis) This is the most common procedure. It is similar to LASEK, but a small flap of the cornea is folded back, rather than removed. It is virtually painless and has the shortest healing time, though you may experience some discomfort, burning, watering, itching and grittiness afterwards. Recovery of vision occurs within a few days, although it may fluctuate for a while and take a few weeks to stabilise. This method is not suitable if your cornea is very thin.

WHATS the EVIDENCE

HOW SAFE IS LASER SURGERY?

Most people undergoing laser eye surgery are very pleased with the results. But there are risks, as with all surgery. According to the Royal College of Ophthalmologists, complications occur in fewer than 5 per cent of cases – although most problems are mild, this is quite a high proportion. They include under-correction, over-correction, infection, dry eyes, glare, haze and a sight-threatening condition called corneal ectasia.

The UK's National Institute for Health and Clinical Excellence (NICE) has pronounced laser surgery to correct refractive errors 'adequately safe and efficacious' in mild or moderate myopia. People who are very shortsighted are less likely to achieve unaided vision; the results are also less good for longsightedness.

your smart sense plan

The book has outlined measures to protect your eyesight and explained how important it is to assess it correctly. If you have less-than-perfect vision, you'll now know that once it's been properly assessed, there are plenty of ways to Correct it – the third step of the PACE strategy, that makes up your *Smart Sense Plan*. You'll be aware of common sight problems, and the importance of regular eye tests. You'll understand precisely why you may need glasses or lenses, how they work, and their benefits and drawbacks, and how surgical procedures can sometimes correct vision defects permanently. It is a good idea at this stage, if you haven't already done so, to write down what you already know about your own sight level, any problems and possible solutions. In the next chapter, you will read about conditions that can still be effectively corrected but might require more specialist medical input.

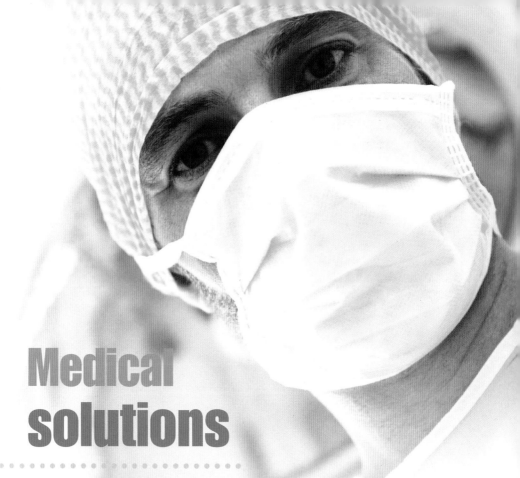

Medical
solutions

4

If you had to choose, which of the five senses would you most fear losing? In surveys, 90 per cent of people say 'sight'. So we are all understandably worried about any disorder that affects our eyes.

The good news is that modern medicine can, if not work miracles, at least do an amazing amount to resolve problems, prevent or even reverse changes, and compensate for any damage already done. In the following pages, you will learn more about the conditions that require medical help and the range of treatments available.

BE ALERT FOR CHANGES

As indicated earlier, eye problems frequently start with few or minimal symptoms and it is important to spot them early so that you can get prompt and effective treatment. It is also true that your vision can deteriorate so gradually that you are barely aware of it.

By remembering the PACE plan – Protect, Assess, Correct and, of course Enjoy this sense – you're more likely to monitor your sight and notice changes as they occur, so you'll be in a better position to take any remedial measures required. Keeping tabs on your eyesight is a continuing, lifelong process – but one which repays the effort with huge dividends.

If a recent eye test has revealed potential problems that will need further investigation, or if you already know that you have, or are vulnerable to, particular eye conditions, then this chapter is especially relevant. And, even if you've been given a clean bill of health, you'll still discover more ways in which you can protect your eyes and guard against future diseases or disorders.

when to seek help

As a general rule, you should consult your optician about any gradual changes in visual acuity (the medical term for how clearly you can see), difficulties with glasses, or symptoms related to wearing contact lenses; see your GP for other eye symptoms or infections. If an eye test has revealed problems that need to be investigated by a specialist, you may need to see your GP for a referral. You'll also be advised to see your doctor if your optician detects changes in your retina that could indicate general health problems such as high blood pressure, high cholesterol or diabetes.

If your eyes are sore for any reason, it will affect your general well-being. For instance, you'll find it harder to read or enjoy watching TV; and you'll probably feel tireder than usual (when your eyes are hurting, all you want to do is close them). So don't suffer in silence. Common eye problems, including eye infections, blepharitis and conjunctivitis (see page 80) or dry eyes (see pages 82–83) can be treated swiftly and easily by your GP, who will also be able to prescribe medication and treat superficial eye injuries.

think**SENSE** ● ● ●

GET HELP NOW!

If you experience any of these conditions, seek urgent medical attention. If you can't get a GP appointment, don't wait; go to a nearby Accident and Emergency or hospital eye department.

- Sudden loss or impairment of vision in one or both eyes.
- Any eye injury.
- A chemical substance in your eye (wash out thoroughly with water first).
- Sudden persistent or severe pain in or around your eye.
- Extreme sensitivity to light.
- Odd visual effects – double vision, halos or rainbows around lights, flashes, black spots or large batches of 'floaters' (see page 23).
- Your pupil is an irregular shape, or fails to respond, dilate or contract.
- Severe redness, itching, burning or watering.
- Profuse greenish or white discharge.

blepharitis – itchy eyelids

If you have dry skin, dandruff or eczema, you may also be susceptible to a common eye condition called blepharitis. This is an inflammation of the inner edge of the eyelids, with blockage of the tiny glands that produce lubricants to help your tear film spread across the surface of your eye when you blink. It can be caused by an infection or an allergy and is not a serious problem. You may notice crusting, scaling and redness at the margins of your lids, and your eyes may feel dry, tired, scratchy, sore and itchy, sometimes with a sticky discharge.

thinkSENSE ● ● ●

DEALING WITH BLEPHARITIS

- Maintain careful hygiene at all times, and wash your face and hair every day.
- Never rub your eyes with your fingers.
- If you wear contact lenses, be scrupulous about keeping them clean and discuss the problem with your optician.
- If you have dandruff, use an anti-dandruff shampoo.
- Avoid eye make-up, or at least try changing to a hypoallergenic brand.
- Always wash your hands before touching make-up or moisturisers.
- Limit your intake of saturated fats and take flaxseed oil (see pages 41–42).

SIMPLE HOME REMEDIES

For crusty and itchy eyelids, try this gentle cleaning option. Soak a flannel or cotton-wool ball in clean hot water – as hot as you can stand without scalding yourself. Hold it over your eyelid for 5 to 10 minutes. Then use diluted baby shampoo to clean the edges of your lids – the lower one first – with a cotton bud or cotton wool. Repeat at least twice a week. If blepharitis makes your eyes feel dry and sore, try lubricating them with artificial tears or lubricating ointment (see page 83). Ask your doctor for advice if you have an associated condition, such as eczema; also see your doctor if you suspect infection or if the condition is really troublesome - you may need an antibiotic ointment or a course of oral antibiotics.

conjunctivitis or 'pink-eye'

Since conjunctivitis gives the whites of the eyes a ghoulish redness, it is widely known as 'pink eye' or 'red eye'. Common in children and older people, it spreads like wildfire in nurseries and playgroups where numbers of children are in close contact and sharing toys. Conjunctivitis affects one or both eyes and is more irritating than painful. Your eyes may also feel gritty, itchy, watery and sensitive to light. Sometimes vision is slightly blurred. You may have a discharge and your eyes may crust over during the night. There are several different types.

It spreads like wildfire in nurseries and playgroups where numbers of children are in close contact and sharing toys.

Infectious conjunctivitis This can be bacterial or viral and may follow a cold or sore throat. Bacterial conjunctivitis tends to cause a thick, yellowish-green discharge and crusting. It usually clears up by itself within a few days, though your doctor may prescribe antibiotic eye drops or ointment. Viral conjunctivitis tends to cause a watery or mucus discharge. It can't be treated with antibiotics but usually clears up in a week or so. Holding a cold compress (such as a wet flannel) to your eyes will help to soothe them.

Allergic conjunctivitis If your eyes are extremely itchy as well as red, the problem may be an allergic reaction. Conjunctivitis that occurs in the hayfever season is called 'seasonal allergic conjunctivitis' and is triggered by pollen or grass. If it happens all year round – prompted perhaps by dust or cat fur – it's known as 'perennial'. Other potential allergens include contact lens solutions, air pollutants, smoke and household aerosols and cleaners. The condition is treated with eye drops, antihistamine tablets or, occasionally, steroid eye drops.

Irritant conjunctivitis Irritation by foreign bodies or chemicals causes a stinging or burning sensation in the eye; there may also be a discharge. Triggers include contact lenses, shampoos and chlorine in swimming pools. Flushing the eye with clean water after a chemical splash is always recommended, but can itself cause this kind of reaction. If a strong chemical, such as bleach or acid, enters your eye, flush it for a good 5 minutes and see a doctor at once. For minor irritants such as shampoo, the reaction should subside in a day or so; if not, see your GP. Avoid eye drops because they could make it worse.

thinkSENSE ● ● ●

STOP IT SPREADING

If you have an infection:
- Wash your hands well and often, especially before and after putting in eye drops or ointment, applying make-up or serving food.
- Don't touch or rub your eyes.
- Change pillow cases, face flannels and towels every day.
- Don't share towels or flannels.
- Stop using contact lenses – use glasses until the symptoms go away.
- Afterwards, throw away any used disposable lenses; clean other lenses and cases thoroughly.
- Replace your eye make-up, especially mascara.

To prevent infection:
- Never share lenses, face flannels, towels, eye make-up or glasses.
- Don't use old eye drops – and never use anyone else's eye drops.
- Wash your hands before touching make-up or moisturisers.
- Don't use old eye make-up or moisturisers.
- Follow care instructions carefully if you wear contact lenses (see page 74).
- Protect your eyes from dirt and other irritants.

dry eyes –
when the tears run out

If your eyes feel tired, irritated and sore after a hard day, or when you've been out in the wind or reading for too long, you may have dry eye syndrome. It tends to happen more as we get older because our eyes produce less moisturising tear fluid, and the tear film itself is less rich in lubricating oils. Other symptoms include itching, slight redness, grittiness and more 'sleepy dust'. Curiously, your eyes may also water a lot in response to irritation– even to the extent of tears running down your face – but these watery tears don't help and will often make your eyes even drier – rather like licking your lips in a cold wind. The good news is that it's easily remedied.

SELF-HELP FOR DRY EYES

Ask your pharmacist about over-the-counter remedies, but if these don't work within a few days, see your GP. Maintaining a healthy lifestyle is good for your eyes in general and helpful for avoiding dry eyes. For example, eating

Eating walnuts and other sources of omega-3 fats is known to be protective.

oily fish, walnuts and other sources of omega 3 fats is known to be protective (see chapter 2), so try to include them in your diet. Or, if you are taking drugs for high blood pressure (medication known to contribute to dry eyes), you can help to lower your blood pressure – and possibly reduce your medication – by cutting down on salt and alcohol, and taking more exercise. And if you don't smoke, you won't suffer the eye irritation that smoke causes, which is also implicated in dry eyes.

TESTING FOR TEARS

Your GP can measure how much tear film you produce by placing a tiny strip of filter paper inside your lower eyelid. After 5 minutes, the strip is examined to see how much liquid it has absorbed.

TREATING DRY EYES

- **Artificial tears** Special eye drops called artificial tears, which keep the eye moist and boost lubrication, help to ease dry eyes. You can get them on prescription or over the counter.
- **Ointment** Use eye ointment to keep your eyes lubricated overnight, but only apply at bedtime as it blurs your vision. If you wear contact lenses, make sure that you take them out before using eye ointment.
- **Surgery** Severe dry eyes can be rectified with one of a range of simple procedures done by an ophthalmologist (hospital eye specialist). Talk to your doctor about this and, if it seems a good option, ask for a referral.

TOP FIVE TIPS TO HELP DRY EYES

- Take regular breaks when doing close-up work, such as reading or sewing.
- Make a conscious effort to blink, and take regular breaks when watching television or using a computer.
- Some conditions or locations make your eyes even drier – sunshine, wind, high altitudes, air conditioning, aircraft cabins, dusty conditions like building sites – so avoid them where possible.
- For the same reason, avoid electric fans; try a home humidifier or stand bowls of water on or near radiators.
- Avoid smoky atmospheres.

when you're referred to a specialist

An ophthalmologist will begin by examining your eyes, either with a hand-held ophthalmoscope of the type used by your optician or with a similar device that uses a hand-held lens and a light attached to a headband, a bit like a miner's lamp. The second method, called indirect ophthalmoscopy, allows a better view of the inside of the eye. The light is much brighter than in an ordinary ophthalmoscope, so you may have more after-images.

PUPIL ENLARGEMENT

For detailed eye examinations, special drops are used to enlarge the pupil and give the examiner a better view. They may sting a little as they go in and cause a funny taste in the mouth (because they mix with tear fluid that drains into your nose and then your throat).

UNIQUE UK EYE CAMERA

One problem with fluorescein angiography is that the dye can trigger an allergic reaction. Thanks to a new British invention, future patients may be able to avoid this hazard. Professor Andy McNaught, a consultant surgeon at Cheltenham General Hospital, has developed a spectral imaging camera that is capable of measuring oxygen levels in the back of the retina, to assess the circulation of the eye and check for glaucoma or diabetic eye disease. And this can be done without the need for dye – or the injection that goes with it.

Be prepared It is comforting to take someone with you to your specialist appointment. You will be told in advance if eye drops are going to be used to dilate your pupils. That is because your vision is blurred for a few hours afterwards and you must not drive. Bring sunglasses too. You may look a bit over-optimistic if it's rainy and overcast, but dilated pupils let in more light than normal and sunglasses will stop you from being dazzled.

TELLTALE PICTURES

A test called a fluorescein angiogram, which also involves dilating the pupils, is used to check for and assess some types of retinal disease. A fluorescent dye is injected into a vein in your arm – and travels rapidly to the eye, where it stains the blood vessels. A series of photographs of your retina, taken with a very bright light, will reveal the state of your retinal blood vessels and give vital clues about conditions such as diabetic retinopathy (see page 98) and macular degeneration (see page 92).

SLIT-LAMP OPHTHALMOSCOPY

The specialist may examine your eyes with an instrument called a slit lamp – a binocular microscope tilted on its side. It's used to investigate disorders related to the outside of the eye, such as corneal abrasions, excessive eye watering, dry eyes, conjunctivitis and eyelid problems, or to look inside the eye for cataracts or other complications that need an enhanced view. You sit in a chair, with chin and forehead resting on supports, looking through a slit, while the specialist illuminates the eye with a variable beam of light from the instrument, which gives a three-dimensional image of the eye.

WHAT A SPECIALIST CAN TREAT

Once you have undergone a detailed examination, you and your specialist will be able to begin planning the best course of action to protect your sight and preserve it in a healthy state. In the next few pages, you will discover which conditions ophthalmologists can treat and details of specific treatments for common sight disorders, including cataracts, glaucoma, macular degeneration (AMD) and retinal detachment.

cataracts –
clearing away the clouds

Less than half a century ago, the onset of cataracts was something to be dreaded because it often heralded blindness. These days, cataracts can usually be cured by a safe, simple operation, performed as a painless outpatient procedure under local anaesthetic. Without exaggeration, this represents a huge and – for sufferers – miraculous, medical advance.

Cataracts are a clouding of the lens, which affects almost everyone over 65 to some degree. The effect is a little like wearing glasses that need cleaning. In the early stages, most people can carry on without treatment and, as outlined in chapter 2, certain dietary changes and vitamin supplements can delay cataract formation. Lens clouding may never become severe enough to need surgery, but it is wonderfully reassuring to know that, if it does, there is a simple remedial operation that really works.

SENSE-sational

WAR INJURIES LED TO CATARACT SURGERY

The procedure for replacing a cloudy, cataract-ridden lens with a clear new one has its roots in incidents that occurred during the Second World War. Pilots returning from combat missions frequently had small pieces of perspex lodged in their eyes from the shattered windscreens of their aircraft. A London ophthalmic surgeon, Sir Harold Ridley, noticed that these did not seem to provoke any reaction within the eyeball – paving the way for the creation of artificial lenses that could be used in cataract operations. He began performing operations soon after the war, and by the 1960s the procedure was widespread.

self-test questionnaire
Spot the signs

Cataract symptoms develop gradually and are painless, so you are unlikely to notice them at first. But if any of the following statements apply to you, see your optician:

☐ The clarity of your sight is deteriorating gradually (over a period of years) – both eyes are affected, though not necessarily at the same rate.

☐ You are increasingly sensitive to bright lights and glare.

☐ You see halos around bright lights.

☐ There are darker patches gradually developing in your field of vision.

☐ There's a brownish-yellow tint to your sight.

☐ Your perception of colour is not as good as it was.

☐ You get double vision in one eye.

BROWN-EYED GIRL

As in other areas of life, there are some risk factors for cataracts that you can't change and others that you can. Those you can't change include being female and having brown eyes. Those that you can do something about include a poor diet and smoking. There are also other factors, which you and your doctor might be able to influence, such as having high cholesterol levels or diabetes, and taking certain medications, such as non-steroidal anti-inflammatory drugs (NSAIDs) and steroids, including inhaled steroids used for asthma. Sunlight exposure used to be regarded as a risk factor, but recently this link has been questioned.

cataract treatment – a modern miracle

About one in five people over 65 and two-thirds of those over 85 develop full-blown cataracts, affecting most of the lens and interfering with vision. Early symptoms may improve with a change in glasses or lens prescription, but in the end, surgery to remove the cloudy lens and replace it with a clear artificial one is the answer, restoring clear vision and the ability to see vibrant colours. It's usually done under local anaesthetic with the help of a sedative. A cataract should be removed as soon as it starts to affect everyday activities such as reading or driving. As a rule, the surgeon operates on one eye first, allowing it to recover before the other is treated. The most common procedure is called phacoemulsification: ultrasound energy is used to break up your own lens, which is then taken out through a small incision and replaced with an artificial lens. It takes about 20 minutes. After the operation you'll need to wear an eye pad for the first few hours. You will be able to see once it is removed, though it may take several weeks for your vision to stabilise. Your surgeon will give you eye drops to help prevent infection and reduce inflammation after the operation.

cutting**EDGE**

MICRO TECHNIQUE

The latest cataract surgery technology can reduce the size of the incision needed to extract a patient's cloudy lens to little more than the size of a full stop. A machine called Stellaris guides the surgeon making the cut, increasing precision, and enables micro-incision cataract surgery through a hole just 1.8mm across. As well as increasing comfort for patients, the tiny wound is self-healing, reducing the risk of infection and focusing problems after the operation, and patients don't need an eye patch. The new device is now being tested in a number of NHS hospitals.

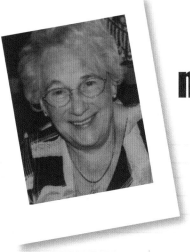

new lens 'absolutely wonderful'

Peggy Sharp

It was only after suffering several falls – breaking both a wrist and an ankle in the process – that Peggy Sharp realised that she had cataracts.

'I just couldn't see properly, but I kept blaming my glasses,' she says. 'It was like looking through mist; I could tell men from women, but not distinguish their faces'. Crucially, she added, 'I couldn't see kerbs.'

> 'I just couldn't see properly, but I kept blaming my glasses'.

Eventually she made an appointment with her optician, who spotted the cataracts and referred her to her GP. She was sent to the local hospital, where she had cataract surgery, first on her left eye, in 2005. She was offered the choice of a local or general anaesthetic and chose to have the procedure under general.

Afterwards, says Peggy, 'It didn't hurt at all. And it was amazing when they took the pad off. I had no idea that my colour vision had deteriorated like that – I couldn't believe how bright the colours were, because I hadn't seen them for so long.'

As sometimes happens after cataract surgery, she developed slight clouding of one eye after a few months. This is due to thickening and clouding of the back part of the lens capsule that is left in the eye to hold the artificial lens in place, and laser treatment quickly resolved the problem. Now in her eighties, Peggy also suffers from acute macular degeneration and needs magnifying aids to read.

> 'It was amazing after the surgery when they took the pad off,' she says. 'I had no idea that my colour vision had deteriorated like that.'

But she is still delighted with the results of her cataract surgery. 'I would say to anyone with cataracts, go and have them done – because it's been absolutely wonderful!'

glaucoma –
early detection can save sight

You may not know you have glaucoma until it is too late. So – perhaps more than any other eye disorder – glaucoma is a dramatic illustration of the importance of regular check-ups. When it is detected early, in most cases it is treatable before any permanent damage is done; undetected, it remains the leading cause of preventable blindness in the UK and the second most common cause (after cataracts) of vision loss in the world. After the age of 40, two in every 100 people has some form of glaucoma; tens of millions of people are affected globally.

ACUTE GLAUCOMA

If your eye suddenly turns red and feels painful, watery and sensitive to light, and your vision is affected to the extent that you see halos, go straight to the nearest hospital's Accident and Emergency department. You might also feel sick and may even vomit.

These are the signs of acute glaucoma, which happens when a sudden obstruction to drainage within the eye causes a rapid rise in pressure. Women are more at risk of the condition than men. Without treatment it can cause blindness, so, even if symptoms begin to ease, you must still go to Accident and Emergency.

LOOSEN THAT NECKWEAR

People with glaucoma who wear tight neckwear may be marginally more at risk of vision loss because of the slight increase in eye pressure. Researchers at the New York Eye and Ear Infirmary tested 40 men, half of whom had glaucoma, before and after they put on a tie to a 'slightly uncomfortable' tightness. After just 3 minutes, they found a significant rise in pressure within the eye in 70 per cent of the healthy subjects and 60 per cent of the men with glaucoma. The pressure fell again as soon as the ties were removed.

The researchers suggest that a tight necktie may constrict the jugular vein, the main blood vessel carrying blood back from the head to the heart, and so lead to increased pressure in the eyeball.

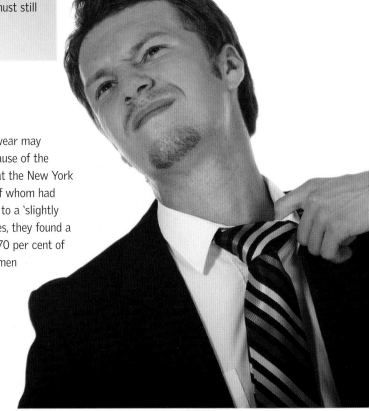

The term glaucoma actually covers a group of eye conditions in which there is damage to the optic nerve that conveys messages from the retina to the brain. The cause is usually a rise in pressure in the fluid contained in the eyeball (known as the intra-ocular pressure) due to the blockage of tiny drainage channels in the anterior chamber of the eye – the compartment in front of the lens.

The risk of glaucoma increases with age; it affects about one in 20 people over the age of 75. Women are at higher risk than men, and if there is a family history of glaucoma or if you are of African origin, your risk is up to four times as great as people who are not in these groups. Other risk factors include being shortsighted or longsighted, and having high blood pressure or diabetes.

UNNECESSARY RISK

Today's techniques mean that 95 per cent of people diagnosed early with glaucoma preserve their sight for life – so never miss an eye test.

Most types of glaucoma affect both eyes, cause no pain and have no other obvious symptoms to begin with. As the pressure in the eye increases, it starts to damage the fibres of the optic nerve, but again, vision loss is so gradual that it is almost imperceptible. Amazingly, we can lose 40 per cent of our vision before we detect any real changes. But by then the nerve damage is irreversible and that vision is lost for good. If it goes untreated, glaucoma eventually leads to tunnel vision – a small area of clear vision surrounded by a dark, blurry 'tunnel'.

THREE TESTS FOR GLAUCOMA

If you are at risk of glaucoma, you are entitled to a free eye test on the NHS every two years, and once you are over the age of 40 the 'puff' test (see page 53) will probably be a part of your regular vision check-up.

cutting**EDGE**

NEW DIAGNOSTIC TECHNOLOGY

A unique new software programme for the detection of glaucoma – which could be made available all over the world, including in developing countries – was unveiled in March 2008 at Moorfield's Eye Hospital in London.

Designed to be effective, affordable and accessible to everyone, the ground-breaking programme can be run on a standard PC or laptop, making it invaluable in the global battle to provide early glaucoma detection.

It is hoped that, once the programme is established, opticians and doctors all over the globe will be able to download the programme from the internet, to use as part of their glaucoma screening services. The software enables clinicians to investigate the visual field (peripheral vision) – one of three recommended assessments in the diagnosis of glaucoma.

After cataracts, glaucoma is the second most common cause of vision loss worldwide. It affects around 67 million people, including some 500,000 people in the UK. As many as 90 per cent of cases in the developing world are undiagnosed.

Appearance of the retina Some changes may be apparent when your retina is examined though an ophthalmoscope, and scans of the retina may be performed, both to check for any damage and to establish a baseline against which to monitor any possible progress of the disease.

Pressure measurement There are several tests, called tonometry, that measure pressure inside the eyeball. These include the puff test and also more accurate tests that involve pressing a small instrument against the outside of the eye and measuring its resistance to pressure. Don't worry, your eyes will be numbed with anaesthetic drops first – but be careful not to rub them until the drops wear off in case you unknowingly hurt them.

Your peripheral vision A test called perimetry looks at what you are able see out of the corner of your eye. You sit with your chin resting at the edge of a bowl-shaped screen, focusing on a light in the middle. Whenever you notice a flash or a movement anywhere on the screen, you press a button; your responses allow the machine to map your visual fields, identifying any areas that you fail to spot. Each eye is tested separately and the whole test takes about 30 minutes.

REDUCING THE PRESSURE

The earlier the treatment is started the better and, in the majority of cases, treatment stops eyesight getting any worse. Most people are given eye drops that control the pressure in the eye, but these are not suitable for everyone; the drugs can cause problems in people who have heart or breathing disorders, for example, and may also interact with medications taken for other conditions, for example, the heart drug digitalis. Laser treatment can also be successful although in some cases, patients need to continue using eye drops. Surgery is an option if other therapies fail.

Overall, drug treatment is successful for most people but you and your specialist might have to try several different types before you find the one that works best for you.

the latest
glaucoma treatments

While drug treatment for glaucoma has successfully prevented vision loss for millions, the drugs are by no means problem-free. Researchers around the world are looking for alternatives – so what might the future hold?

ALZHEIMER'S DRUGS?

In 2007, researchers at University College London discovered that beta-amyloid, the protein that builds up in the brains of people with Alzheimer's disease, is also deposited in retinal nerve cells when pressure in the eye increases. When the team introduced beta-amyloid into the retinal cells of rats, it provoked glaucoma-type damage, which may explain why Alzheimer's sufferers are at risk of the same kind of visual impairment as found in glaucoma. The team then tested (again, on rats) experimental Alzheimer's drugs that aim to stop beta-amyloid accumulating, and found that they reduced the death rate of retinal nerve cells in eyes with glaucoma. Other research shows that drugs used in Alzheimer's as nerve protective agents may also prevent damage to the optic nerve from raised pressure in the eyeball – but none has yet been approved for treating glaucoma.

cutting**EDGE**

LOW-FREQUENCY LASERS

A new type of laser surgery appears to offer a quick and relatively painless treatment for open-angle glaucoma (the most common type) and may be especially helpful for people whose condition has not responded well to pressure-lowering eye drops. The procedure – selective laser trabeculoplasty (SLT) – makes it possible for lasers to be operated at very low frequencies and to treat specific cells in the drainage system of the eye on a selective basis, lowering intraocular pressure. As untreated areas of the eye around the iris are unaffected, SLT – unlike other types of laser surgery – can be safely repeated many times. It takes less than a minute per eye and is available at an increasing number of UK centres.

ANECORTAVE ACETATE (RETAANE)

A single injection of this drug – a modified steroid, initially proposed as an AMD drug – may be able to control pressure in the eyeball for three months or more, according to research presented at the 2007 World Glaucoma Congress in Singapore. Clinical studies are underway and, if they are successful, the drug could be launched as early as 2009.

GLATIRAMER ACETATE (COPAXONE)

This drug given by injection for multiple sclerosis has so-called 'neuroprotective' effects that could translate into protection for the optic nerve against the effects of glaucoma.

macular degeneration
or AMD

Sometimes described as a 'disease of civilisation', AMD is a condition in which the cells in the macula begin to deteriorate. Since it usually occurs in older people, it is commonly known as age-related macular degeneration – hence the AMD acronym. Luckily, retinal changes can be seen in an eye examination long before vision is impaired, so regular eye tests could save your sight. And there is plenty you can do to protect your eyes from AMD, from stopping smoking to getting regular exercise and adopting a healthier diet (see page 38).

(see page 38).

THE EFFECTS OF AMD

If it is left untreated, AMD will result in the gradual loss of your central vision – making detailed work much more difficult – and the loss of colour vision.

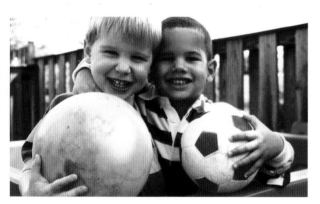
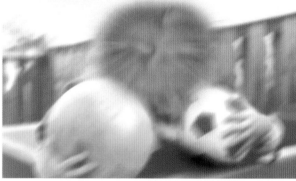

AMD causes initial blurring and then gradual vision loss from the centre outwards as the central part of the retina thins. Research in the *Journal of the American Medical Association* in April 2007 found that common variations in two genes, together with smoking and obesity, greatly increased the risk of the disease progressing.

Experiencing the loss of colour vision is likened by some people to watching the colours fade in an old photograph. It does not cause total blindness, because your peripheral vision is unaffected. This means that you can still get around independently, but you will eventually lose the ability to read, write and drive a motor vehicle.

SPOTTING THE SIGNS

Like many eye conditions, AMD is painless. It usually affects both eyes, although one may be affected long before the other. Since the 'good' eye compensates for the failing one, AMD can remain undetected for years. The trouble is, that by the time you become aware of deteriorating sight, your chances of successful treatment have faded significantly.

The earliest symptoms include difficulty focusing on detailed tasks such as reading or sewing, blurred vision, and what are in fact straight lines appearing wavy or fuzzy in the centre of your field of vision. Colours may look less bright, and it may be difficult to recognise small objects or distinguish faces straight ahead. Eventually, you may become aware of a blank patch or dark spot in the centre of your vision.

WHAT CAUSES AMD?

Scientists don't yet know why some people get AMD and others don't, but they think that a mixture of genetic and environmental factors is involved. There is a higher risk in people with a family history of the condition, and there is an inherited form that affects children and young people called macular dystrophy. Some scientists think that free radicals – by-products of the metabolism of cells, which can damage DNA – may play a role in AMD. The intense metabolic activity in the macula produces lots of free radicals, and if these are not neutralised – by, for instance, antioxidant vitamins and minerals in foods – they could slowly damage the cells of the retina. This may also explain why sunlight and radiation seem to speed up macular decay. See pages 38–44 for protective foods.

cutting**EDGE**

NEW KNOWLEDGE ABOUT AMD

In the past few years, several independent studies have found two gene variants, known as complement factor H (CFH) and complement factor B, that are strongly associated with AMD. CFH increases the risk of developing AMD, but there is not much point in genetic testing, since as many as 38 per cent of us carry the CFH gene, yet few of us will go on to develop AMD.

But CFH is involved in regulating inflammation – and blood levels of a marker of inflammation called C-reactive protein (CRP) have been found to be raised in people with AMD. So the discovery may assist future research into the prevention and treatment of inflammation underlying the development of AMD. Researchers are now searching for the specific triggers that set off the immune response – and subsequent inflammation – but suspect that it will take from seven to ten years before any cure for AMD is in sight. .

TREATMENT FOR AMD

AMD occurs in two forms, 'dry' and 'wet'. In dry AMD – by far the more common form – small areas of fatty deposits called drusen accumulate in the retinal cells under the macula. They make the macula thin, leading to

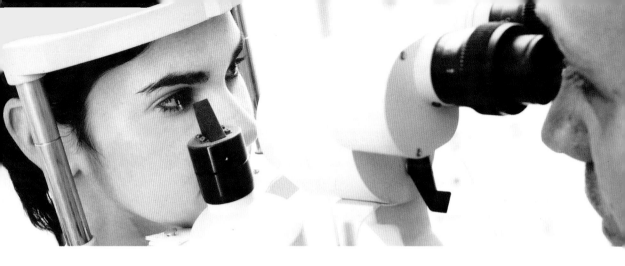

Keep up to date with your eye tests, since dry AMD can develop into the more serious – but treatable – wet form.

gradual impairment of central vision. Fortunately, dry AMD develops slowly and the changes are usually quite mild, rarely leading to total loss of vision. At the moment there is no treatment for dry AMD, although researchers are investigating whether antioxidant vitamin supplements might slow down its progression. And, needless to say, it is worth eating a healthy diet. You must also keep up to date with your eye tests, since dry AMD can develop into the more serious – but treatable – wet form.

Only 10 to 15 per cent of cases of AMD constitute the more aggressive wet form, in which tiny, fragile blood vessels develop under the macula. These then leak behind the retina, causing scarring and damage to sight in a matter of weeks or months. Blind spots appear in the centre of the visual field and gradually become larger until eyesight is virtually destroyed. But if wet AMD is identified at an early enough stage of development, one of the following treatments may slow down or even reverse the damage.

Photodynamic therapy (PDT) Suitable for only a minority of patients, photodynamic therapy involves injecting a light-sensitive drug into the arm. The drug travels through the bloodstream to the blood vessels in the eye, showing up the abnormal ones. A low-energy 'cold laser' is then beamed into the eye and activates the drug, which destroys the vessels without harming surrounding tissue.

Relocation of the macula Surgical relocation of the macula is a very specialised operation that is suitable for relatively few AMD patients, but it has a reasonably good record of success.

Anti-VEGF therapy This relatively new treatment is based on drugs that inhibit a protein called VEGF (vascular endothelial growth factor), which is involved in the formation of new blood vessels in the macula. The drugs,

practical performance test
Spot the early signs of AMD

You can take a basic test for AMD – the same one that professionals use – at this very moment. It is called an Amsler Grid and it can detect some alterations in central vision (used for reading and other close work) before you spot them. You can also use this to track any changes if you already have AMD.

Warning: This test is no substitute for a professional eye test. Only an expert can diagnose AMD or other conditions that affect central vision (and so may influence the test). But if you do notice any of the effects described, make an appointment to see your optician straight away.

How to take the test
- Make sure the room is well lit.
- Hold the page at your normal reading distance – which should be about 40cm (15in) away from your eyes – wearing your reading glasses or bifocals if necessary.
- Cover one eye (but don't close it or press on it).
- Focus with the other eye on the black dot in the middle of the grid and stare at it fixedly for about 20 seconds.
- Note what you see, then repeat the test with the other eye.

See page 96 for an analysis of the results.

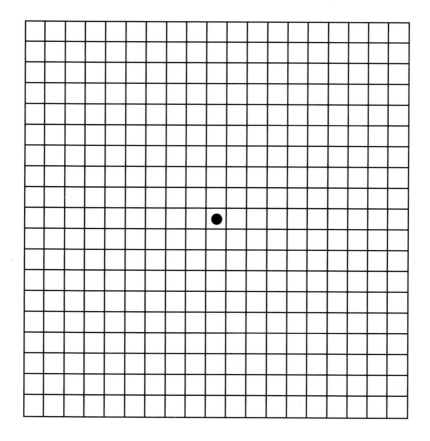

Results

- If you see straight vertical and horizontal lines, parallel and evenly spaced, forming a grid with evenly spaced, identical squares – like graph paper – then your central vision is probably normal. Congratulations. All you need to do is to carry on having regular eye tests every two years or as often as your optician recommends.
- If you see horizontal and vertical lines that are at any point crooked, wavy or distorted, or if there are any gaps in the lines, or the lines bend inwards towards the black dot at the centre, or some of the squares are a different size or shape to the others, or there is any blurring or discoloration over the grid, then you may have altered central vision. This is important to know as you may have identified an eyesight problem in time to stop further damage. Make an appointment to see your optician straight away.

cuttingEDGE

STEM-CELL TECHNOLOGY MAY CURE AMD

In future, patients with either form of AMD may have the prospect of a complete cure, thanks to groundbreaking research sponsored by the London Project to Cure Blindness. The project director, Professor Pete Coffey of University College London Institute of Ophthalmology, is leading a team of scientists who have successfully implanted human stem cells into the retinas of pigs – a vital first stage in their quest to replace degenerated macular cells in people with AMD. The team has already shown that cell-replacement therapy can work in principle in humans using patients' own cells. Stem cells are far more adaptable, and they believe the technique will be 'capable of stabilising and restoring vision in the vast majority of patients who currently suffer blindness through AMD'. Clinical trials in people could begin within the next five years.

which are injected into the eye, reduce the growth of new leaky blood vessels. Treatment is carried out under the close supervision of a consultant ophthalmologist and needs to be repeated every one to six weeks for up to two years.

BREAKTHROUGH TREATMENT

Anti-VEGF therapy has dramatically changed the outlook for patients with wet AMD. It halts the deterioration of sight in more than 90 per cent of patients; in about a quarter of cases eyesight actually improves, suggesting that treatment can reverse existing damage.

At the moment, there are two drugs licensed for the treatment of AMD in Britain: Lucentis (ranibizumab) and Macugen (pegaptanib). Lucentis seems to produce better results than Macugen. In two major international trials, most patients who were treated with Lucentis retained a visual acuity within three lines of their baseline on a Snellen chart (see page 56). Even more startling, about one-third of treated eyes had near-normal visual acuity (Snellen 6/12 or better), an outcome that the *British Medical Journal* described as 'unattainable' with previous treatments.

But the drugs are very expensive and not universally available on the NHS. Hope lies in a ground-breaking, NHS-funded trial which will compare Lucentis with another, much cheaper drug called Avastin (bevacizumab), from which Lucentis was derived, which seems to have similar effects. The results will not be available for several years, but some doctors do offer Avastin 'off label' for AMD; it is currently used to treat some types of cancer.

retinal detachment –
a medical emergency

Retinal detachment is a condition in which the retina comes away from the back of the eye. This rare event, which affects only one in 20,000 people each year, can be successfully treated to prevent damage to eyesight – as long as it is identified at an early stage and treated quickly. In recent years, two British prime ministers, Margaret Thatcher and Gordon Brown, have suffered from the condition.

In most people, retinal detachment is preceded by the detachment of the vitreous humour (the gel in the back of the eye), leading to a hole or tear in the retina. This causes a sudden onset of painless, brief but bright flashes in the periphery of the visual field, with sudden showers of floaters. Most vitreous detachments, however, do not damage the retina, and many tears do not progress to retinal detachment.

CURTAIN ACROSS THE EYE

Sometimes, however, a tear allows fluid to seep underneath the retina, so that the retina peels away in the manner of stripped wallpaper, creating a sensation like a shadow or curtain being drawn across the eye. Straight lines may look curved – door frames may appear to bend, for example. Eventually, central vision is lost and, if the entire retina becomes detached, it can cause blindness. Fortunately rapidly administered treatment can stop the detachment and halt the process.

Vitreous detachment can be caused by trauma, such as a squash ball or tennis ball scoring a direct hit or a punch to the eye – so pursuits such as boxing are obviously risky, and boxers should have frequent eye tests.

The risk of retinal detachment increases with age, and is also raised in people with diabetes and those who have had cataract surgery. Very shortsighted people have a lifetime risk of about 1 in 20 (15 times that of a normally sighted person) since their longer eyeballs mean that the vitreous humor exerts a greater pull on the retina, while the retina itself is stretched and thinner than normal.

MENDING THE TEAR

Holes or tears in the retina can be repaired with laser or cryotherapy (freezing) to stop them progressing to full-blown detachment, and this is successful in most cases – although between 5 and 9 per cent of patients will have another tear in future.

Even if detachment has started, the retina can be reattached using various forms of surgery involving heating, freezing or lasers; about one in five people treated will need more than one operation. Eyesight might be blurred for several months and treatment may not restore full vision. If the detachment affects the macula, central vision could be permanently damaged. About one in 20 people suffer a second detachment.

diabetic retinopathy – eye tests essential

People with diabetes, which affects more than 2 million people in the UK, are especially vulnerable to a number of eye complications. They are more likely to be shortsighted, or longsighted, or colour-blind, and may be prone to eyelid infections, early cataracts and dry eye syndrome. Diabetes doubles your risk of glaucoma, and increases the risk of macular disease and retinal detachment. In addition, diabetics are especially susceptible to a condition called retinopathy, where the retina becomes damaged as a result of high blood sugar levels. Keeping your diabetes under control reduces the risk of complications substantially, and for many diabetic eye problems there are effective treatments.

WHAT SYMPTOMS?

One of the most worrying aspects of diabetic retinopathy, which can cause severe sight problems or loss, is that in the early stages there are seldom any symptoms, so regular eye tests – every six to 12 months – are essential

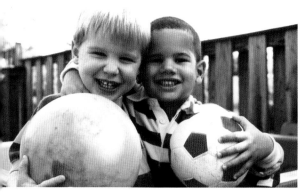

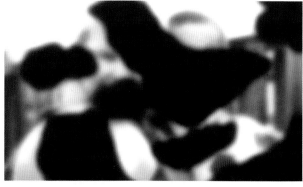

Normal vision

Same scene viewed by someone with retinopathy

- to detect changes before any damage occurs. In the UK, people with diabetes are entitled to free NHS eye tests. Untreated, other symptoms will occur as the diseases advances. These include:

- spots in front of your eyes
- dark streaks or a red film that affects your sight
- a deterioration in your night vision
- blurred vision and loss of vision

Retinopathy usually affects both eyes and is likely to be worse the longer you have had diabetes and the less stable your blood sugar control. In the early stages there may be swelling and later blockage of some of the tiny blood vessels of the retina. Eventually new blood vessels are formed – so-called 'proliferative retinopathy'. These grow along the surface of the retina and, as in macular disease, are abnormally fragile. If they leak, this can obscure vision and may lead to blindness.

Smoking 20 cigarettes a day triples your risk of retinopathy, and simply being exposed to other people's smoke can double your risk.

RISK FACTORS YOU CAN CONTROL

Anyone who has diabetes is vulnerable to retinopathy. But there are other risk factors that you can influence. For instance, the risks are highest if you are not controlling your blood sugar well, if you have high blood pressure and if you have high cholesterol. Smoking 20 cigarettes a day triples your risk of retinopathy, and simply being exposed to other people's smoke can double your risk.

For the sake of your eyes and the rest of your body, work with your GP and specialists to keep your blood sugar, blood pressure and fat levels under control. Have regular eye tests, keep to a healthy diet

NATIONAL PREVENTION PROGRAMMES WORK

Active regular screening and standard laser therapy can be highly effective in controlling diabetic retinopathy, according to the health authorities in Iceland. A national diabetic eye screening programme was started there in 1980 and appears to be working well to prevent blindness and partial sight loss in people suffering from Type 1 and Type 2 diabetes. The programme was reviewed over a four year period. Of the 205 patients who participated initially, 175 stayed with the programme, receiving eye tests and appropriate laser treatment. The sight of 7.4 per cent of the subjects improved by two Snellen lines (levels on the standard eye chart), while 2.5 per cent experienced some deterioration. The review reported that in Type 1 diabetics participating in the programme, vision levels remained stable and the incidence of retinopathy was 'low'.

(see pages 38-44), keep your salt levels low as this influences blood pressure, and try to take at least 30 minutes' exercise every day.

RETINOPATHY TREATMENT

Laser treatment can slow or even stop the disease progressing and will normally be recommended if you have proliferative retinopathy. This is usually carried out in a darkened room in a clinic. Anaesthetic eye drops are administered, a contact lens is placed on your eye and you sit at a laser slit lamp, which flashes a highly focused, bright light or series of lights onto the side or 'periphery' of your retina. Your vision may be blurred for a day after the treatment and your eye may ache for a few days. You may also notice spots in your side vision or see flashes of light at night.

Laser surgery is almost always successful, but it may require several treatments and possibly further treatment at a later stage. It is not a complete cure because diabetes is a lifelong condition, so future retinal damage can occur. Researchers are working on new treatments, such as medications that can be injected into the eye to treat abnormal blood vessels or even prevent them from forming.

your smart sense plan

As this chapter explains, most common eye conditions – such as dry eyes and conjunctivitis – can be diagnosed and remedied by visiting your GP. These conditions may be irritating and can temporarily impair your vision, but they won't usually damage it.

With more serious eye conditions, as outlined above, it is essential to have regular check-ups and to seek help as soon as you detect any symptoms. However worrying the diagnosis, there is almost always something that can be done to help. The treatment of eye conditions is improving all the time, while the future of vision research is one of the brightest hopes in medicine.

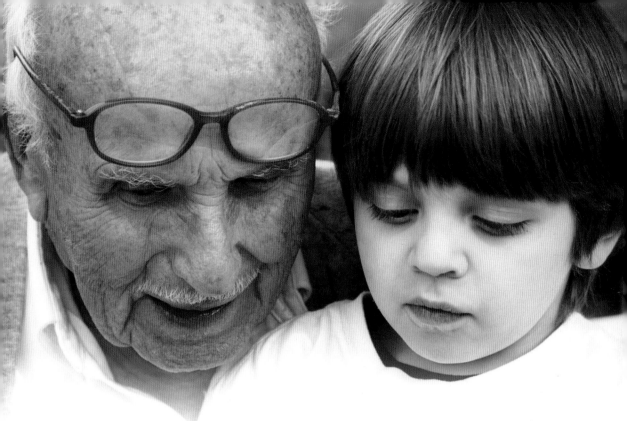

5   The wider picture

We all want to see as well as we can for as long as we can – for the joy of welcoming new family members and appreciating all the beautiful things around us. But, once you start tackling eye problems and correcting them – by getting the right lenses or glasses, or whatever it takes to boost your vision – you will probably realise that you need to make small adjustments in your life.

If your vision isn't perfect, you need to make a few changes to ensure that everyday life is easier, safer and more enjoyable. In this chapter you will learn some practical strategies that will help you to compensate for less-than-perfect eyesight.

Even if your own sight is currently perfect, these are things you'll want to know if you or a loved one ever suffers any future vision loss. It's another form of 'correcting' and an integral part of your *Smart Sense Plan*, which is all about seeing the best you can and getting as much pleasure as you can from your eyesight – for life.

HEALTHY EYES, HEALTHY BODY

The healthy-living strategies that form part of your *Smart Sense Plan* could save your life as well as your sight, as many of them will also help to protect against common causes of premature death, such as heart disease and some cancers. That is a good reason to pursue a healthy lifestyle even if you have continuing vision problems. And, if you follow the advice in this chapter, you will help to protect yourself from two other major hazards – road accidents and falls.

TAKE ACTION

Impaired vision does not have to affect your quality of life unduly as long as you are prepared to keep assessing your sight, adjusting your lifestyle as required and taking advantage of every advance in optical science that you can. A number of studies have shown that, unfortunately, older people frequently don't wear glasses when they should or are using out-of-date prescriptions. Many don't realise that their vision is getting worse and are unaware of the importance of regular eye tests. Now that you're following your *Smart Sense Plan*, that won't affect you. But if, despite professional help and your own best efforts, you still have problems, there are numerous ways in which you can compensate.

watch your step

Trips and falls – often caused by something we misjudge or fail to see – are always a shock to the system. But, as you get older and your bones get more brittle, you are more likely to break something in a fall – perhaps a wrist or hip, which could have a lasting effect on your quality of life; hip fracture is the most common cause of permanent loss of independence among elderly people. Because deteriorating vision is one of the main causes of falls in older people, it is especially important to have your eyes tested regularly, to keep your lens prescription up to date, and to replace your glasses if they get scratched.

SIGHT AND BALANCE

Eyesight is important for our sense of balance. Visual clues about body position and movements in our surroundings help the brain to stabilise the body. That is why a shifting environment – which misleads the brain about where everything is – causes seasickness, and why you are less likely to be able to stand up straight if you close your eyes. So-called 'postural sway' increases by between 20 and 70 per cent when people close their eyes while standing upright. Not surprisingly, then, poor vision increases sway and reduces balance.

practical performance test
How good is your balance?

Here is a simple test you can do at home: the one-legged balance test. You will need a stopwatch or an observer with a watch that has a second-hand.

- Wearing flat shoes or in bare feet, stand up straight facing a counter or a sturdy high-backed chair (to grab onto if you start to wobble). If you are in any way uncertain about your balance, take the test only if you are standing by a bed as well – and preferably with someone else around to catch you in case you fall.
- Fold your arms across your chest and raise one leg, bending it at the knee at an angle of about 45°. Close your eyes and at the same time start the stopwatch or ask your observer to start timing you.
- Stop the clock as soon as you uncross your arms, become unsteady or need to put your other foot down. Give yourself a couple of minutes' break, then repeat the test with your other leg.

Check your time compared with age-group averages:
20 to 49 years old: 24 to 28 seconds
50 to 59 years: 21 seconds
60 to 69 years: 10 seconds
70 to 79 years: 4 seconds
80 and older: most people cannot do it at all

If you are well below the average time for your age group, think about doing some balance-training exercises, and check with your GP whether any medications you are taking or any health problems could be interfering with your balance. It is a good idea to repeat the test periodically.

CONTRAST AND DEPTH

It is not only our ability to read small print that deteriorates as we age. There is also a reduction in something called 'contrast sensitivity', which makes it harder to distinguish the outline of different surfaces so we may not detect hazards such as kerb edges and steps, especially in dim light. Studies have shown that this blurring effect is more likely to be the cause of a fall than a simple reduction in sharpness of vision. Depth perception is even more important – in one study it proved the strongest predictor of falls out of nine different measures of vision. Depth perception relies on two eyes working together; if you have good sight in only one eye, your risk of falling is as high as people with lesser vision in both eyes.

UP THE WOODEN HILL

When it comes to the causes of trips and falls, stairs are a prime culprit. But they don't have to be. Make sure that the stairs in your home have proper handrails fitted on both sides. These must be strong enough to bear

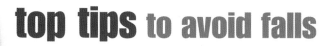

top tips to avoid falls

Did you know that at least a third of all falls in older people happen at home? And that they usually involve something as obvious as tripping over a loose rug? Just as parents of toddlers are urged to crawl around looking for danger spots, it can be a good idea for adults to 'walk the walk' around the house and garden, in good daylight, spotting potential hazards.

Here are some obvious ones:

- Loose objects on floors or pathways
- Trailing electric and telephone cables
- Slippery floors and baths
- Rickety furniture
- Worn carpets, especially on stairs and landings
- Poor lighting
- Loose rugs
- Poorly placed furniture, such as low coffee tables
- Lack of adequate hand-holds on stairs and in bathrooms

But there are plenty of easy ways to make your home safer

- Keep floors tidy – remove all stray objects and find places to store them.
- Move or tape down electrical flexes and cables.
- Arrange furniture to give a clear path in and out of rooms.
- Get rid of oversized or awkward furniture that obstructs movement; foot stools are a notorious trip hazard.
- Remove castors from furniture feet or put castor cups under them to stop the piece of furniture from rolling around.
- Use carpet tape to anchor rugs securely – or get rid of them.
- Mend or replace worn and loose carpets.
- Put down anti-slip mats in bathrooms and in front of the kitchen sink.
- Use an anti-skid mat in the bath or shower, and a non-slip bath mat on the bathroom floor if it's uncarpeted.
- Install any shower shelf at a sensible height so that soap or shampoo are easy to reach; many people slip in the shower while bending to retrieve a dropped item.
- Fix handles and grab rails in the bathroom, on stairs and on outside steps.
- Don't polish or wax solid floors.
- Install adequate lighting both indoors and out, especially near stairs or steps.
- Ask a friend or relative to inspect your outdoor space for possible dangers each spring. Make sure that paths are kept free of moss, plants, leaves, garden implements, stones and other debris; and replace or repair cracked paving slabs and uneven walking surfaces.

think**SENSE**●●●

SHOE WISDOM

If your eyesight is not as reliable as it used to be, always wear well-fitting, low-heeled shoes. Even if they are your most comfortable footwear, worn-out shoes or slippers should be replaced before they become a tripping hazard.

your weight and securely anchored to the wall, so it's a good idea to get a professional to install them.

Brightly coloured self-adhesive tape applied to the edge of each step will make it easier to see, and if you use contrasting colours on the first and last steps you can easily see when you get to the change of floor level at the top or the bottom of the stairs.

Have a telephone beside your bed, so you don't have to rush downstairs to answer it, or use a cordless phone or mobile, and keep a torch nearby in case of power cuts.

LIGHT FANTASTIC

People can be curiously unconcerned about reducing dangers in their home. It is obvious that life is easier, more comfortable and far safer if you can see what you're doing. So don't put up with dismal dark corridors and spooky staircases. Have more lights installed. But make sure that the type of illumination you choose is appropriate – some 'green' energy-saving bulbs light up very slowly, which can be a hazard. Equally, the wrong type of illumination that glares or dazzles you is almost as bad as no light at all. And electric light is no substitute for daylight. Here are a few bright ideas.

- Make sure that doorways, stairs and passageways are well lit with bulbs of the maximum appropriate wattage.
- Leave landing or hall lights on overnight in case you need to leave the bedroom.
- Ensure you have light switches within easy reach at the top and bottom of stairs and at both ends of corridors.
- Have sufficient lights throughout the house – make sure kitchen surfaces are well lit, and add table and floor lamps in living areas if fixed lighting is poor.
- Avoid bare bulbs, clear-glass shades and chandeliers that can produce glare and dazzle.

SENSEalert

MULTIFOCALS CAN MULTIPLY THE PROBLEMS

If you are at an age when turning 40 is a distant memory, or you are at risk of falls or fractures for other reasons, you need to think carefully before choosing multifocal (bifocal, trifocal or varifocal) glasses or contact lenses. These are made to aid distance vision at the top of the lens and near vision at the bottom of the lens. The trouble is that they impair both distance contrast sensitivity and close-up depth perception – a double disadvantage that can reduce your ability to spot looming hazards at ground level.

Many studies show that multifocals increase the risk of falls among older people, some of them indicating that wearing such lenses makes a fall more than twice as likely. So think about using a single lens prescription for distant vision plus a set of reading glasses. If you want multifocals for, say, computer work, then take them off before you walk around the house, especially to walk up or down stairs, and don't wear them when going out, especially when travelling on public transport.

Continued on p108 ▶

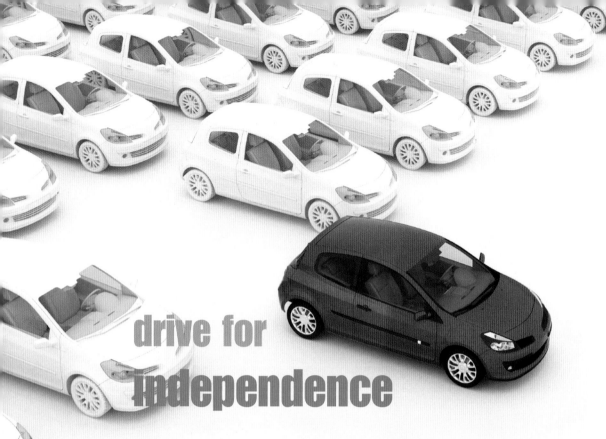

drive for independence

Some eyesight changes that occur as we get older can affect our driving ability. For example, it gets harder to refocus when viewing distant, then close-up, objects. Reaction times are slower and you need more light to see.

It also becomes more difficult to adapt to very bright light, particularly to sudden dramatic changes in light intensity – emerging from a heavily tree-lined road into the sunshine, for instance. Peripheral vision tends to worsen and colours may be dimmed. But there are many steps you can take to mitigate these problems:

- Don't drive when you are tired.
- Stay alert and concentrate. Make sure that there is a good flow of air through the vehicle and take frequent breaks.
- Always wear your glasses or lenses if you need them for driving; keep your glasses clean.
- Keep your windscreen clean inside and out.
- Wear good-quality sunglasses in bright light. Be aware that low sun can produce excessive glare and 'bleach out' white road markings so that they are difficult to see; glasses can be treated with an anti-reflective coating to reduce glare.

- Avoid glasses with wide side-pieces and wrap-around sunglasses, since they may block your side vision.
- Keep pace with the speed of other cars, but don't drive too close to the car in front.
- Take extra care at junctions and crossroads, especially when turning right.
- Consider an older driver's assessment check (see box) or even an advanced driving course (see Resources, page 238).

DRIVING AFTER DARK

Many people over the age of 40 find night driving increasingly difficult. Our eyes adapt more slowly to dim light and are more sensitive to glare and dazzle. The most obvious solution is to plan journeys to avoid dusk and night time. If that's not possible, the following tips will help your night driving, irrespective of your age:

- Keep to well-lit main roads if you can.
- When you know that you will be driving at night, avoid bright sunlight during the preceding day. The brighter the light and the longer your eyes are exposed to it, the longer they will take to adapt to the dark. So in daylight wear sunglasses or a wide-brimmed hat, and stay in the shade as much as possible. But don't wear any sort of tinted glasses when you drive at night.
- Make sure that your headlights are properly adjusted for the best forward illumination.
- Opt for an anti-reflective coating on your glasses, to reduce glare.
- Drive more slowly at night, keeping to a speed that allows you to stop within the distance lit up by your headlights.

EYESIGHT, DRIVING AND THE LAW

If it is some considerable time since you passed your driving test, you must notify the Driver and Vehicle Licensing Agency (DVLA) if you develop certain visual problems.

You DON'T need to tell them about:

- Shortsightedness or longsightedness, if correctable by glasses or lenses.
- Colour-blindness.

You DO need to tell them about:

- Any other visual disability which affects both eyes.

think**SENSE**●●●

POLISH YOUR DRIVING SKILLS

SAGE (Safer Driving with Age) is a programme designed to enhance the safety of mature drivers or those returning to driving after a period off the road. It is offered at low cost by many local councils. SAGE includes a check to confirm that medications and vision are not impairing your driving, followed by a one-hour driving assessment with an experienced assessor. It is not intended as a test. The programme is based on common sense and safe, skilful, everyday driving, with no trick questions or unusual manoeuvres. It is conducted in your own car and on familiar roads. You can discuss your driving performance and will be given a confidential written report afterwards.

The Institute of Advanced Motorists offers a short driving assessment, called DriveCheck, aimed at people who want reassurance about the safety of their driving. It is friendly and informal, and, again, it is not designed as a pass/fail test.

NIGHTLIGHT FOR NIGHT SIGHT

This advice contradicts something you read earlier in the book (see page 64). If you're at risk of falls, the hazards to your safety of reduced night vision far outweigh the benefits of sleeping in the pitch dark. So do use a nightlight – the ones that plug into wall sockets are affordable and widely available – so you don't come a cropper if you need to go to the bathroom. And take one with you if you're staying away from home. If you forget, ask your host if you can leave a landing light on, or if you're in a hotel leave the light on in the bathroom all night and the door ajar.

- For reading and desk work, use freestanding lamps (task lighting) that can be raised, lowered and swivelled. Keep the light behind and to one side of your working area, so that it is shining downwards onto what you're doing.
- If your colour perception is less good than it was, you can buy halogen or fluorescent bulbs that are designed to improve colour rendering; ask a lighting retailer about the options.
- Where light switches are hard to see or to reach, consider installing motion-sensitive lighting that switches on automatically when you enter a room; check that the light will stay on for a comfortable period of time.
- For outdoor safety, install automatic motion-sensitive lights on driveways, paths and outside doorways.

BOLD AND BEAUTIFUL

Generally, strong contrasts make objects easier to see. So if you keep tripping over the sofa, try covering it in a boldly coloured fabric or painting the wall behind it a contrasting colour. Put striped borders around your light switches so they're easier to see in dim light. But minimise contrast in lighting between rooms since your eyes will find it hard to adapt quickly. For the same reason, give yourself a moment or two to adjust if you come indoors from a sunny garden or go out into the sun from a dark room.

little helpers

There are all sorts of things that can make daily life easier for partially sighted people. These aids can make such a difference to your quality of life that you will be much less conscious of any sight problems you have. Here is a small sample of what's on the market. If you want to discover more, look at the Resources section on pages 238-239.

- Choose watches and clocks with huge numbers and thick hands, and avoid Roman numerals, which are harder to distinguish.
- Look for large-print books at your local library.
- Computer keyboards are available with large keys and big letters set against different-coloured backgrounds, as well as touch pattern keys.

when strawberries are green

People who are colour blind (see pages 54-55), don't simply see the world in black and white, of course. But they may find it almost impossible to distinguish between certain colours. Here are some tips for dealing with a few of the practical difficulties of colour-blindness.

- Fluorescent light can disguise even colour differences that you might normally distinguish, so when buying clothing or decorative household items, take them to a window or outside (after checking with the shop assistant first).
- If you are red–green colour-blind, you may not be able to detect skin reddening – so put on plenty of sunscreen in sunlight so that you don't end up lobster pink.
- Is it hard to tell when meat is cooked properly? Don't try to judge whether food is cooked solely by its appearance; instead, always follow recommended timings, remembering to preheat the oven. Best of all, ask someone else to confirm that food – especially pork and chicken – is properly cooked.
- Buy some sock locks. Everyone has the problem of odd socks appearing from the washing machine, but if you are colour-blind you may never match them up again. Sock locks are little plastic rings that bind socks together when you take them off so they go straight through the washing machine and back into the drawer as a pair.
- Look for computer software that allows you to detect and adjust colours on screen, including colours on web pages.

- Set the text size on your word processor to large and experiment with different colours and backgrounds – often yellow text on a black background is easier to read than black on white.
- Choose felt tips rather than biros to write with.
- Voice-recognition software can interpret what you say and transform it into written form; speech software that translates printed text and reads it back to you is also available.
- Specialist suppliers have an astonishing range of products for people with visual impairment: large-print calendars, talking or tactile watches and clocks, magnifiers for reading and writing, and writing frames to help you to write straight and sign cheques in the right place.
- You can obtain voice-activated mobile phones, talking books, audio-set timers, talking thermometers and liquid-level indicators.
- You can even get a hand-held CCTV camera to capture and magnify images wherever you are, for instance to read the very small print on supermarket labels.
- Remember, too, that service providers are legally obliged to provide large-print bills, statements and other crucial information.

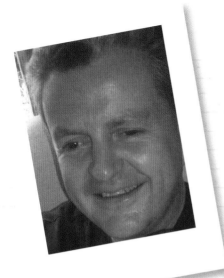

Embracing the challenges

Simon Meredith

Simon Meredith is a successful corporate tax lawyer, a trustee and co-founder of a registered charity, and the father of two young children. He has also been blind since the age of 13.

'I had perfect eyesight until I was 12,' he remembers. 'Then one May bank holiday weekend I developed a sudden pain in one eye. My sight in that eye disappeared over three days.'

Tests were conducted and doctors diagnosed an unusual eye condition – optic neuritis (inflammation of the optic nerve) – but as his other eye worked well he went back to school and normal life. Six months later, while playing rugby, he suddenly realised that a road sign beyond the playing field was blurred. The sight in his other eye gradually deteriorated over the next six months to the extent that, at the age of 13, it was accepted that he needed special education, and he went to a boarding school for blind children.

> 'I had perfect eyesight until I was 12, then one May bank holiday weekend I developed a sudden pain in one eye.'

At that stage he could still see enough to find his way around, and even to kick a football and read with a magnifying glass – but not well enough to recognise faces. But by the age of 14 he had lost most of the sight in his second eye, and he had to learn to use Braille to read. Now, he says, 'I can't see anything'. It's not black, though. 'There are lots of brightly coloured red, green and purple dots, and they change a bit – but I don't really notice them any more. Occasionally I get a bit of light and movement in the periphery – I can sometimes tell where a window is, but that's about it.'

A STEEP LEARNING CURVE

At school Simon was given mobility training, learning how to detect obstacles ahead and use non-visual cues such as sounds and the texture of the ground to get around; as a result he can travel independently. 'There are ways to orientate yourself when walking', he says. 'You get to know a familiar area – you can tell by the smell when you walk past a fish shop, or a wine merchant, or even a newsagent.' He's never had a guide dog and uses a cane to get about, taking public transport including the London Underground. 'You can hear what's going on', he says. 'You can tell the flapping noise of the ticket barriers, and if you stand and listen you can detect when a member of staff is nearby from the sound of their walkie-talkies. Staff are well-trained; they know how to say "Do you need assistance?" in a neutral way. There's a lot of help available if you know how to access it.'

Even so, he has to plan ahead, find out where the nearest tube station or dropping-off point is, and how to get there from where he's going on foot. 'Sometimes going somewhere new is just too much trouble,' he admits. 'Some days just stepping out of the front door and walking down the road takes too much effort. But if you don't embrace challenges like that, you'd stay inside all your life.'

WHAT TECHNOLOGY CAN OFFER

Simon is now assessing new Wayfinder Access software that enables blind and visually impaired people to use GPS (satellite navigation) technology relayed to a mobile phone, with an earpiece and a voice-driven menu. If you put in the postcode of your destination, it will walk you there (it can also establish your precise location).

Working in a complex area of tax law, Simon uses a lot of modern technology. He has the JAWS screen reader and speech output software on his laptop to enable operations in audio mode, and a Braille Lite notetaker for diary, address book and document functions in Braille, along with Talx speech software to enable use of all the functions on a standard mobile phone. 'I'm a telephone junkie', he says. 'I'm so paranoid about losing one that I have three mobiles, just in case.'

'I lead a very normal life in many ways,' says Simon, 'but I've spent a lot of money on technological aids and being able to employ someone to help with paperwork and administration. Not everyone is able to do this.

'Losing your sight is very frightening, but the only way to combat the fear of the unknown is to find out what's available – get as much information as you can.' Many people end up dependent on local social services networks that can be very variable, often lack continuity, and may not have full knowledge of what's possible.

'Losing your sight is very frightening, but the only way to combat the fear of the unknown is to find out what's available

That is why ten years ago, with two friends who are also blind law graduates, Simon set up 'Blind in Business', a registered charity to help blind and partially-sighted people to identify and achieve their ambitions. It helps young people through education and on to good careers via employment and training services, offers help to mature job seekers and to employers thinking about taking on visually impaired workers. 'The staff are knowledgeable about all the equipment and opportunities available, helping blind and partially sighted people to lead a rich and fulfilling life,' says Simon.

(For contact details of Blind in Business and other organisations, see Resources, page 238.)

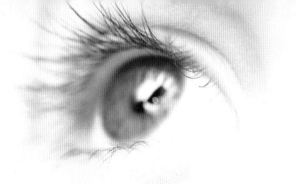
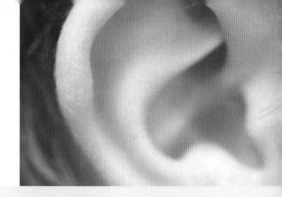

6 your smart sight plan

No two people have identical eyes or exactly the same sort of vision. So, whatever plan you devise for yourself will be as individual as you are, based on what you now know about your eyesight and your particular concerns. We hope that you are much more aware of your eyes than you were: how they work, what can go wrong, how professionals can help, and what you can do to maintain your vision in the best possible health for the rest of your life. **Here is a quick summary to help you check that all the** PACE **elements of your** *Smart Sense Plan* **for optimum eyesight are in place.**

Protect your eyes

- Are you overweight? 31, 44
- What sort of sunglasses do you wear? 32
- Do you sleep in darkness? 32, 64
- How often do you take a break when you're doing any kind of close work? 33
- How long do you spend under artificial light each day without a break? 34
- Do you wear goggles when drilling or doing other risky DIY jobs? 35
- Have you followed our eye-protective guidelines for computer work? 36-37
- Do you know what an eye-healthy diet looks like? 38-44
- Have you ever considered taking supplements? 45
- Do you smoke? 46-47

Assess your vision

- Are you finding it more difficult to see in the dark? 26
- Are you increasingly dazzled by headlights when driving at night? 26
- When did you last have an eye test? 49
- How good is your colour vision? 54-55
- On the 20/20 scale, how sharp is your eyesight? 56-57
- Have you made a note of your eye test results? 57
- Do you have any vision symptoms or difficulties? 58-67
- Do you know what glaucoma is? 88

(Keep track of any changes with time - this is a continuing plan.)

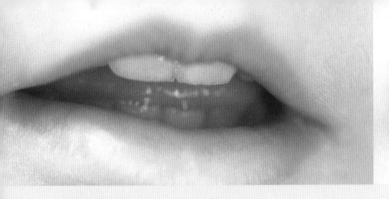
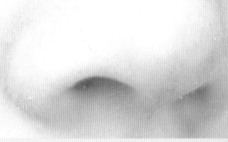

Correct any problems

- Do you know which eye conditions are emergencies, when you should seek urgent advice, if necessary from an Accident and Emergency department? 79
- Do you ever have tired, scratchy, sore and itchy eyes? Do you know how to treat them? 80
- What precautions should you take if you or a family member has conjunctivitis (also known as pink eye or red eye)? 80-81
- Do you suffer from dry eyes? If so, have you consulted your GP? 82-83
- Are you frightened of cataracts? If so, don't be. Discover how your eyesight can be saved. 85-87
- Did you know that 95 per cent of people diagnosed early with glaucoma keep their sight for life? It's worth an eye test – especially if you are over 40 or have a family history of the disease. 88-91
- Have you taken our basic eye test for macular degeneration? It's no substitute for professional advice. If you have any concerns, see your optician. 92-95
- Do you know why you must rush to the doctor if you ever experience bright flashes of light and showers of floaters? 97
- If you have vision problems, have you tried any of the 'little helpers' that make life so much easier? 108-109

Enjoy your sense of sight

- Remember the sights and scenes that make you really happy.
- What's your favourite colour?
- Where is your favourite view? Can you picture it?
- And where in the world do you dream of visiting? Extraordinary places of great natural beauty, perhaps, or man-made wonders.
- Think about the faces of all the people you love. You probably know every tiny detail.
- What do you enjoy most about your home or garden? It's probably the colours and shapes that come to mind.
- How do you like to relax? Reading, watching films or television, walking in the countryside? Your eyes are your guide.

If you imagine not being able to enjoy these things, it will give you all the incentive you need to look after your eyes.

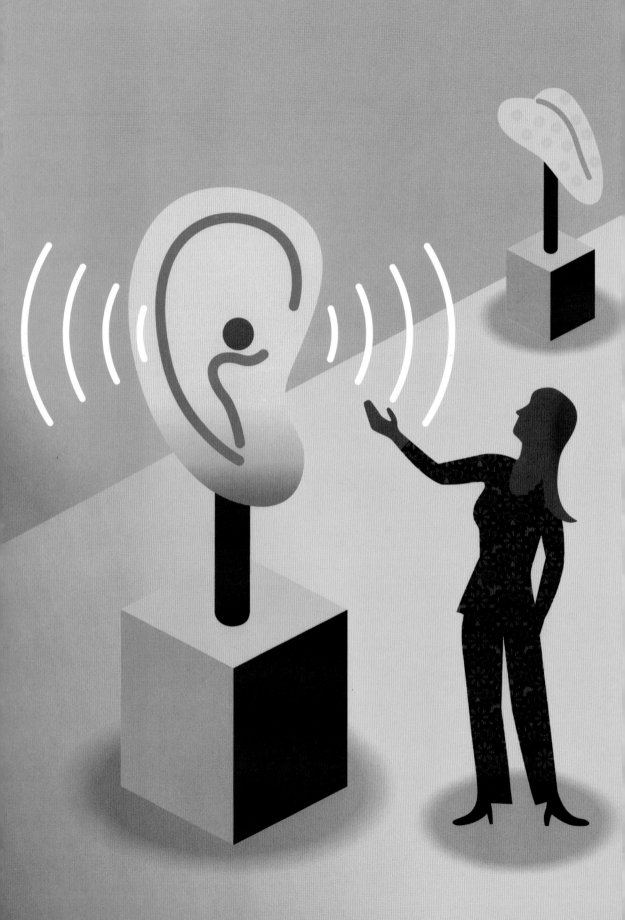

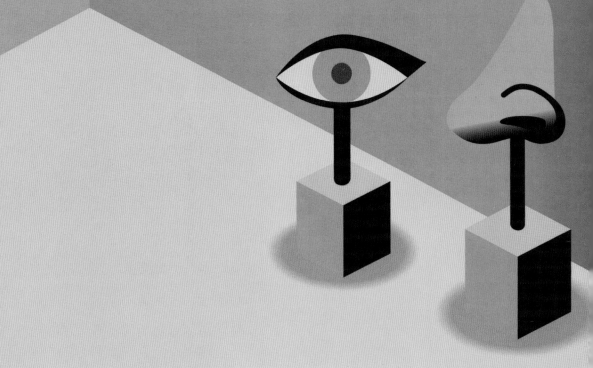

Hearing

We live amid a cacophony of daily noise
but, as we get older, many of us find that some sounds –
such as the telephone ringing – become more difficult to
hear. Fortunately, as you will learn in this section, there
are many ways to prevent and overcome such problems,
so you'll be able to enjoy conversation, music and all the
sounds you love for years to come.

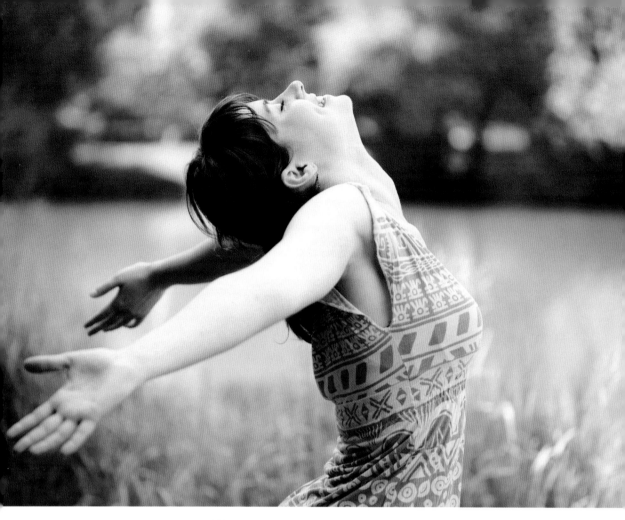

7 The joy of hearing

What would the world be like without sound? All of us can imagine to some extent what it would be like to be blind – we simply have to shut our eyes. It's much more difficult to imagine being unable to hear speech or music or the dawn chorus, or even the clatter when you drop a pan or your own 'ouch' when you stub a toe.

There may be sounds that you would rather not hear – the throbbing music leaking from a fellow passenger's headphones, the road drill outside your office window, the car alarm that goes off at two o'clock in the morning, your next-door neighbour's lawnmower disturbing a lazy summer afternoon in the garden … yet wouldn't it feel strange if you *couldn't* hear them?

self-test questionnaire
Have you got a hearing problem?

Do you have difficulty hearing or following what is being said in the following situations?

☐ Listening to the television when the volume is adjusted to suit someone else.

☐ Talking on the telephone.

☐ Having a conversation with someone in a busy place, such as a street, shop or restaurant.

☐ Having a conversation with several people in a group.

☐ Listening to someone against a background noise, such as a whirring fan or running water.

☐ Having a conversation when you can't see the other person's face full on.

☐ Talking to women or children – even though you can hold conversations with men without any difficulty.

Do you often:

☐ Ask people to repeat what they've said?

☐ Misunderstand what people say?

☐ Agree or nod even when you're not sure what's been said?

☐ Feel that other people mumble when they talk?

☐ Turn up the radio or television to a volume that others say is too loud?

☐ Have to watch other people's facial expressions or lip movements to understand what they say?

The world is, by and large, such a noisy place that relative calm and silence – which are important for our general well-being – have become rare treats to be relished. But as we get older, the world may become uncomfortably quieter if certain important sounds are more difficult to hear – for instance, the telephone ringing, a grandchild crying, or the best moments of a favourite symphony.

Even minor degrees of hearing loss can cause intense frustration – when you have to strain to hear what other people are saying, miss crucial spoken information such as station announcements, or feel left out in social situations because you can't follow conversations if there's a lot of background noise.

Yet, even if a certain amount of hearing loss is inevitable as we grow older – and it's by no means certain that it is – there is much that can be done to protect this vital sense and there are many causes of hearing loss that can be treated. In this section you will learn all about your ears and the remarkable process of hearing. You will find out why balance disorders may result from ear problems and about other symptoms, such as tinnitus

A ROCK CONCERT IN YOUR CAR?

Did you know that some of today's in-car stereo systems are capable of producing more volume than the speakers used to provide sound for a whole stadium during a Beatles or Rolling Stones concert in the 1960s?

(a persistent, irritating sound in the ears), which can accompany them. Because you're concerned enough about your senses to be reading this book, you will no doubt want to take steps to preserve your hearing and your enjoyment of the sounds of life – for life.

MEASURING SOUND LEVELS

Sound is measured in decibels – a term derived from the Latin for 'ten' plus the name of Alexander Graham Bell, the inventor of the telephone, and shortened to dB. Any sound-measurement scale has to include a huge range of sound intensities, from a ticking watch to a jet aircraft taking off – a difference of 200,000,000,000 times – so scientists use a logarithmic or 'log' scale, which means that every increase of 10dB represents a sound that is ten times as loud. Whether noise causes hearing loss depends both on the intensity of the sound and the length of exposure.

it's a loud, loud world

In towns and cities the sound often never stops. Many people must endure constant noise from traffic, even at night, and loud sounds are everywhere: emergency sirens, power tools, car alarms, burglar alarms, building works, lawn mowers and leaf-blowers. There is no escape. That's not to mention the ear-splitting volumes to which we expose ourselves for pleasure, such as thumping in-car stereo sound systems, nightclubs and rock concerts. Scientists are in no doubt that exposure to excessive noise can be harmful to our hearing.

It usually takes a long period, between 25 and 30 years, for noise-related hearing damage to accumulate. However, as a result of the increasing din of modern life, and especially exposure to loud music and portable music players, hearing specialists are now seeing increasing numbers of young people with 'old ears'.

Many people must endure constant noise from traffic.

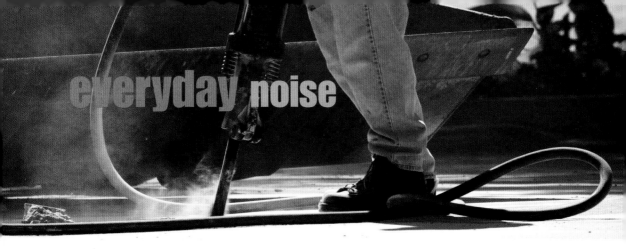

everyday noise

On the decibel (dB) scale, 0dB is near-total silence, but 10dB is ten times more powerful, 20dB is 100 times more powerful, 30dB is 1,000 times more powerful, and so on.

A hair dryer at 80dB is a hundred times as loud as normal speech at 60dB. A rock concert booming out at 120dB is a million times as loud as normal conversation.

Decibels (dB)	Sound
0	Near silence
20	Ticking watch, rustling leaves, quiet room at night
37–45	Computer hum
50–65	Dishwasher, washing machine
60	Normal conversational speech

Intrusive

65	Average city traffic

Difficult to concentrate

70	Television, busy office, noisy restaurant, vacuum cleaner

Annoying

80	Hair dryer, alarm clock, heavy traffic, shouting

Hearing impairment on prolonged exposure

84	Train
85–90	Leaf blower
90–95	Lawn mower, busy pub
90–100	Motorcycle
95–140	Loud car stereo
100–120	MP3 portable music player

Painful even on brief exposure

110	Chain saw, pneumatic drill, nightclub/disco, baby crying
110–120	Ambulance siren, jet aircraft on take-off
130	Thunderclap, machine gun

Possible irreversible hearing loss

119–140	Heavy-metal rock band
164	.357 Magnum pistol

45-YEAR-OLD EARS AT THE AGE OF 15

In fact, today's young people have a rate of impaired hearing two-and-a-half to three times greater than that of their parents and grandparents. An average 15-year-old may now have as much hearing damage as an average 45-year-old, and experts are predicting an epidemic of hearing impairment as today's teenagers gets older.

Also, of course, a vicious circle is eventually created. As more people experience hearing difficulty, more sounds in public places have to be turned up to a level that the 'average' person can hear, for example in the cinema. The earlier you take action to protect your hearing the better – and you will find plenty of advice on how to do so in the next chapter. But, whatever your age, you can start to protect the hearing that you still have and enhance its quality.

ONE IN SEVEN

As we live in a world full of noise pollution, we often don't appreciate just how important hearing is to us. Many people are unprepared for hearing loss until something happens to alert them to the problem – but it affects around one in seven people in the UK and becomes increasingly common as we get older.

More than one in three people aged over 50 and more than half of those aged over 60 have some degree of hearing impairment. Most forms of hearing loss can be prevented, treated or alleviated; there is no need to suffer in silence. But since hearing loss tends to creep up on us slowly, it is all too easy to be unaware of what we are missing. And if we don't realise when we have a problem, we miss out on the help that's available.

In chapter 8 you'll learn how your lifestyle can help you to preserve your hearing. You'll find out how to check if you have any symptoms that might suggest a problem, and the various medical causes of hearing disorders and how they can be treated. And in later chapters, you'll discover how modern hearing aid technology is transforming lives.

SENSE-sational

UNNATURAL NOISE

If our ears are designed to detect and interpret sound, why is it that noise can be so harmful? Surely, being sensitive to noise is what ears are for? Well, not quite. Our ears evolved to pick up biological sounds, not the roar of engines and the din of amplified electronic sound. Our remote ancestors needed to hear relatively quiet noises that could be crucial for survival, such as the approach of a wild animal that could be hunted for food or might be intent on eating you. The loudest sound was probably the odd thunderclap, and even occasional loud noises were interspersed with long periods of relative silence.

how we hear

Sound travels through the air as waves of vibration that are detected by the ears and converted into electrical impulses. These impulses are sent by means of nerves to the brain, which decodes the signals to interpret the sounds. The process bears some resemblance to the way in which light is detected by the eye and converted to electrical impulses that enable the brain to process images.

Although sound detection involves a number of intricate and delicate structures in the inner ear, the mechanism is fairly straightforward. First, your outer ear – the visible fleshy part – collects and funnels sound waves down the ear canal leading to the eardrum. This is more important than

your hearing equipment

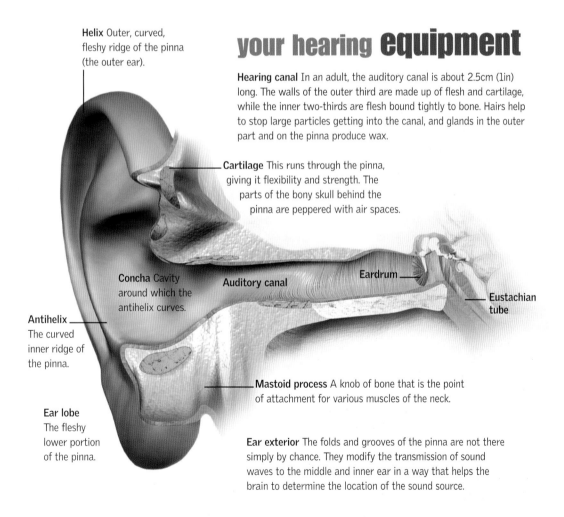

Helix Outer, curved, fleshy ridge of the pinna (the outer ear).

Hearing canal In an adult, the auditory canal is about 2.5cm (1in) long. The walls of the outer third are made up of flesh and cartilage, while the inner two-thirds are flesh bound tightly to bone. Hairs help to stop large particles getting into the canal, and glands in the outer part and on the pinna produce wax.

Cartilage This runs through the pinna, giving it flexibility and strength. The parts of the bony skull behind the pinna are peppered with air spaces.

Concha Cavity around which the antihelix curves.

Auditory canal

Eardrum

Eustachian tube

Antihelix The curved inner ridge of the pinna.

Mastoid process A knob of bone that is the point of attachment for various muscles of the neck.

Ear lobe The fleshy lower portion of the pinna.

Ear exterior The folds and grooves of the pinna are not there simply by chance. They modify the transmission of sound waves to the middle and inner ear in a way that helps the brain to determine the location of the sound source.

it sounds: unlike most other mammals, we cannot adjust the position of our ears to hear noises that could spell danger, such as the sound of an approaching predator. The drum itself – known technically as the tympanic membrane – is a thin sheet of tissue that separates the outer from the middle ear, and vibrates when 'hit' by sound waves. On the other side of the drum, the middle ear contains three tiny bones – called ossicles – in a linked chain, bridging the gap between the drum and part of the inner ear called the cochlea. The snail-shaped cochlea consists of a spiral tube filled with fluid. Vibrations of the drum are amplified by the ossicle chain and transmitted to a small 'window' in the cochlea.

the middle ear

A tiny tube called the Eustachian tube links the middle ear to the back of the nose and throat, ensuring that the air pressure in the cavity stays the same as the pressure outside it. During sudden changes in external pressure, such as when an aeroplane lands, the pressure inside the ear often cannot be equalised fast enough, leading many people to complain of earache. This effect is especially common in young children, whose tubes are smaller than those of older children and adults. Yawning, sucking or chewing helps to open up the tube – which is why air crew may offer boiled sweets to passengers before a plane begins its descent – and why the feeling of fullness in the ear after a flight often disappears with a satisfying 'pop'.

The Eustachian tube also admits air, helping to drain any secretions that build up in the middle ear, for example when an infection is present. Blockage of the Eustachian tube by conditions such as colds or sinusitis can lead to the unpleasant bunged-up feeling that often accompanies respiratory infections and may cause sounds to be temporarily muffled.

SENSE-sational

YOUTH GANGS ENCOURAGED TO BUZZ OFF

A gadget that exploits youngsters' ability to hear higher frequencies than their elders has been developed to dispel gangs of loitering teenagers. The 'mosquito' is a sonic deterrent that works by emitting an extremely irritating noise that older people can't hear. The intensely shrill ultrasonic tone, which is harmless, becomes increasingly annoying the longer it is heard – but generally only those under 25 receive the full impact; for older people it's a mild buzzing sound.

The device has a range of 15 to 20m (50 to 65ft) and, in many areas, has been so successful at stopping youths congregating that some police forces are investing in it as a means of decreasing vandalism, antisocial behaviour and criminal damage (though civil liberties groups, who object that the devices indiscriminately target all young people, including babies, have called for a ban).

Meanwhile, one enterprising youngster has turned the buzz into a mobile-phone ringtone, so teenagers can hear their phones ringing without adults – such as teachers or parents – knowing.

Check your hearing

How is your hearing coping with the cacophony of the modern world? If you want to do a quick self-assessment, you can take a simple hearing test either by telephone or online. According to the Royal National Institute for Deaf People (RNID), 4 million people in the UK are losing their hearing and not doing anything about it. Don't be one of them.

- To take a RNID telephone hearing test, call 0845 600 5555*. The test takes less than 5 minutes. You will be asked to key in your age and gender, then listen to a series of three-digit numbers played against a rushing background noise. After each number – 4 3 9, say, or 2 7 8 – you key in what you hear. At the end of the test you get an immediate result and information on where to go for help if you need it.
- If you have a computer with a soundcard and headphones, try a free online test, such as: www.siemens-hearing.co.uk/uk/05-about-hearing/02-hearing-loss/01-hearing-test/hearing-test.jsp

*Calls to 0845 numbers cost more than those to 01 or 02 numbers, and can be expensive from mobile phones.

inside the inner ear

The vibrations are transmitted in turn through the fluid in the cochlea, where they are detected by tiny hair cells. There are more than 15,000 of these hair cells, from which, as their name suggests, tiny hairs, called cilia, protrude. The hairs move in response to vibrations and generate electrical signals – rather like pressing the keys on an electric piano keyboard. The signals are transmitted through the auditory nerve to the brain, where they are interpreted as meaningful information, whether in the form of speech, music or the ticking of a clock.

HIGH NOTES, LOW NOTES

Different hair cells respond to different sound frequencies (a frequency is determined by the number of sound vibrations that are generated per second). High-pitched noises, such as the top notes of a violin or a soprano singer, create more vibrations per second than low-pitched ones, such as the sound of a tuba or a deep voice.

The hair cells in our ears that respond to high-frequency sounds seem to be more vulnerable – they are the ones most likely to be damaged by noise, and the ones that are lost first as we get older. That's why people with hearing loss often have trouble with women's and children's voices but can hear men quite clearly. It's also why young people can hear high-pitched sounds that older people can't, and why high-pitched noises are most damaging to our hearing.

IS HEARING LOSS INEVITABLE?

Most medical professionals believe that age-associated hearing loss, known as presbyacusis, is to an extent inevitable. But studies of a Sudanese tribe called the Mabaan, who live in quiet rural surroundings, show that they have much better hearing than Westerners – indeed, even older members of the tribe have better hearing than 20-year-olds living in industrial societies. What's more, among the Mabaan there is little difference between the hearing of young people and the tribal elders.

Apart from their quieter life, the Mabaan people's excellent hearing may be influenced by their diet – a factor discussed in the next chapter. Meanwhile, all the evidence seems to suggest that it is well worth protecting ourselves and our children from the potentially deafening effects of loud noise.

HAIR TRIGGERS

The hairs in the cochlea can respond to minute vibrations – they need to be moved less than the diameter of an atom to produce a signal, and can detect pressure variations of less than one billionth the level of atmospheric pressure. But the vibrations produced by loud noises create much bigger pressure waves, which damage the hairs by bending them too far.

If the hairs are damaged, the hair cells die off – and, since they cannot be replaced, this can eventually lead to permanent hearing loss. Loud noises may also impair the blood supply to the hair cells and to the auditory nerve, leading to the formation of scar tissue that stops the cells functioning properly. And recent research has shown that excessive noise provokes the formation of more free radicals – damaging chemicals that build up in cells during metabolic functions and contribute to ageing and decay. This too can cause permanent damage to the hair cells and to the auditory nerve.

a question of balance

The inner ear is also crucial to our sense of balance. The reason that ear disorders often cause dizziness and balance disorders as well as hearing loss is because our balance-control mechanisms are so near the organs of hearing in the inner ear.

The vestibular or balance organs inside the inner ear include three fluid-filled circular tubes, called the semicircular canals, positioned at right-angles to each other. These detect rotational movements in any direction by sensing disturbance of the fluid within them. In addition, the part of the inner ear known as the vestibule contains tiny granules that are displaced during head movements, which detect gravity and movement in a straight line. All this is contained in a minute structure not much larger than a dried pea. Each inner ear has its counterpart in the other ear. The brain senses any discrepancy between the signals from the two ears

Ear disorders often cause dizziness and balance disorders as well as hearing loss.

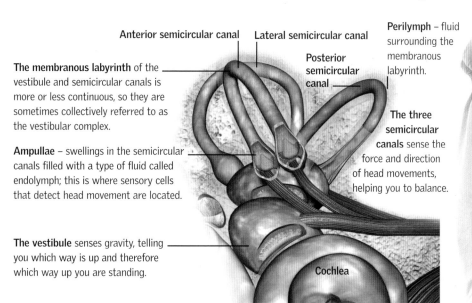

Anterior semicircular canal

Lateral semicircular canal

Posterior semicircular canal

Perilymph – fluid surrounding the membranous labyrinth.

The membranous labyrinth of the vestibule and semicircular canals is more or less continuous, so they are sometimes collectively referred to as the vestibular complex.

Ampullae – swellings in the semicircular canals filled with a type of fluid called endolymph; this is where sensory cells that detect head movement are located.

The three semicircular canals sense the force and direction of head movements, helping you to balance.

The vestibule senses gravity, telling you which way is up and therefore which way up you are standing.

Cochlea

and interprets that as movement. It then sends instructions to our eyes and joints to make compensatory adjustments to keep us balanced so that we don't topple over.

WHEN THE BRAIN'S IN A SPIN

The brain also receives sensory input from the eyes, joints, skin, muscles and spinal cord. When everything works properly, we have a remarkable ability to sense the direction we're facing, which way is up, whether we are still or moving, turning or straight, and in what direction we are heading. But any conflicting messages between different parts of the system can literally send our brain into a spin. That's what happens when you are seasick or when you are affected by inner ear disorders.

your smart sense plan

This chapter contains some vital facts about hearing to help you with your *Smart Sense Plan*. Importantly, you've learned how even the noises of everyday life can cause slow, insidious damage to hearing – but that hearing loss need not be an inevitable part of ageing. In the next chapter, you'll learn how to Protect your hearing (the first step of your PACE strategy) from harmful influences such as noise, and other ways to preserve this precious sense for as long as possible, and perhaps even enhance it.

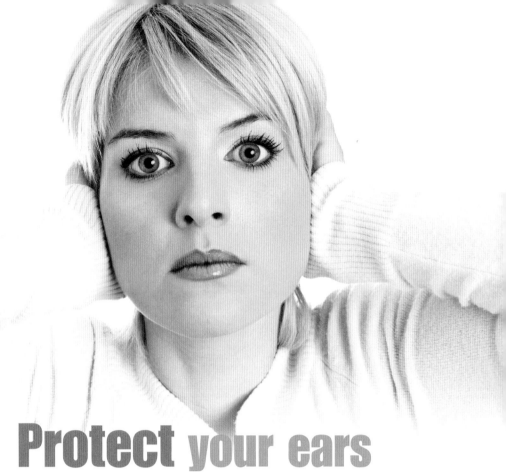

8   Protect your ears

Even if you did spend rather too much of your youth listening to rock bands at full blast, there is still plenty you can do as part of the Protect stage of your Smart Sense Plan to guard your ears from continuing noise assault and minimise any further loss.

Several other factors are important for the health of your hearing – from adopting a well-balanced diet to effective treatment of ear infections – and there are other ways to keep your hearing as good as it can be as you grow older. Experts estimate that, worldwide, as much as 50 per cent of hearing loss is preventable.

NOISE CAN DAMAGE YOUR HEALTH

First, it is worth identifying and being aware of the elements of modern life that can threaten good hearing. This will not only help you to protect yourself against hearing loss and tinnitus (persistent, irritating sound in the ears) by reducing the noise levels in your environment, but also allow you to shield yourself from distraction and get a better night's sleep.

Prolonged exposure to noise makes people tired and irritable; noise in the workplace increases accident rates and makes it harder for workers to relax and unwind at the end of the day. It's been estimated that as many as half a million people in the UK have hearing problems as a result of noisy jobs – which means that the number suffering from noise-related stress is probably even higher. Noise can create learning problems for schoolchildren and students and stimulate aggression. Unwanted background noise has been shown to increase the level of cortisol, a stress hormone, that is excreted in urine. High noise levels have been associated with increased headaches, heartburn, indigestion, stomach ulcers and a type of dizziness known as vertigo.

A study by Johns Hopkins University in Baltimore showed that noisy hospital environments slow down the pace of healing in patients and cause short-term memory lapses; they also increase the risk of medical errors and lead to higher stress levels among staff.

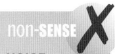

non-SENSE

EARS ADAPT TO LOUD NOISE

A myth has taken hold that regular exposure to loud noise can 'toughen up' your ears so that the noise won't bother you any more. But if you believe that you're getting used to a regular attack on your hearing, what's actually happening is that you're going deaf! The reason it doesn't affect you as much as it used to is that you have already lost some of your hearing – so take action to protect yourself before you lose any more.

NOISE AND HEART DISEASE

Noisy environments are related to increased heart rate, blood pressure and blood cholesterol levels, and there is a growing suspicion that noise may contribute to heart disease. The World Health Organization warns that long-term noise exposure above 67 to 70dB (equivalent to moderate traffic noise) can lead to high blood pressure, raising the risk of cardiovascular disease. Studies have shown that even moderate noise over a single 8 hour period can increase your blood pressure significantly.

Other research suggests that exposure to noise above 50dB during the night can lead to chronically raised cortisol levels that may increase the risk of heart attacks. Anything above 45dB is likely to interfere with sleep. Both high blood pressure and cardiovascular disease have been linked with increased rates of hearing loss.

In fact, the detrimental effects of noise are so widespread that some campaigners in the USA are calling for 'secondhand noise' – intrusive sounds produced by other people – to be treated as a health hazard just like the passive inhalation of secondhand cigarette smoke. The European Environment Agency says that about 65 per cent of people in Europe are exposed to ambient sound at levels above 55dB, while about 17 per cent of us live with noise above 65dB. These levels may not seem exceptionally high – they simply represent the sounds of everyday life made by, for example, air and road traffic, human speech, radios or domestic appliances – but if you are subject to prolonged exposure, even 'normal' levels of this kind are unacceptable.

HOW NOISY IS TOO NOISY?

Sensitivity to noise varies from person to person, so how can you tell if you are being harmed? You may be damaging your hearing if:

- A noise hurts your ears.
- You use heavy power tools for more than 30 minutes daily.
- You are exposed to regular impact noises, such as hammering or pneumatic drills.
- Continuous noise – from, for example, being in a crowded public place, working in an environment that includes noisy machinery or living close to a busy road – is intrusive for much of your day.
- You experience ringing in your ears during or after noise exposure.
- The quality of your hearing is reduced in the hours after exposure to loud noise.

SENSEalert

SPLIT-SECOND TRAUMA

As well as the steady drip-drip effect of continuous noise pollution leading to gradual damage to your hearing, it is possible to suffer immediate and sometimes permanent hearing loss from a single exposure to a very intense noise, such as a bomb blast or gunshot at close range. It takes a very loud noise – in the region of 140dB – to cause such harm, but the damage can be done in as little as a fifth of a second. Known as acoustic trauma, the pressure wave of a blast physically damages the inner ear. Sometimes it can burst the eardrum or even damage the tiny ossicle bones in the middle ear as well.

BLOCK YOUR EARS

Acute hearing loss resulting from very loud noise, whether a sudden blast or exposure over several hours (standing next to loudspeakers at a rock concert, for example), sometimes clears up over the following couple of days – but sometimes it does not. So an important step in protecting your hearing is to avoid sources of very loud noise that can cause damage in a short time – and persuade others, especially young people, to do the same. Major culprits include industrial machinery, power tools, building sites, clubs and discos, concerts, firework displays, close proximity to aircraft (for example, if you work at an airport), loud music and farm equipment. When you cannot avoid loud noise, limit your exposure to the shortest time possible, wear ear protection (earplugs or ear defenders), and if you are obliged to endure being surrounded by sound over prolonged periods, try to give your ears a rest at regular intervals – 10 minutes every hour, say.

HOW EARPLUGS BECAME COOL

Many people who grew up during the 1960s and 1970s, when music amplification became widespread, paid no attention to the sensitivity of their hearing and are now living to regret it. Some of the most acclaimed performers of the period, including Who guitarist Pete Townshend, Neil Young and Sting, and others who were musicians and audio engineers at the time, now have significant hearing loss. Luckily, we are now alert to the dangers of noise, and these days musicians and DJs are much more likely to wear earplugs when working or playing.

PLUG IN, TUNE OUT!

Hearing experts are genuinely concerned about the effects of portable music players such as MP3s and iPods. According to the RNID, two-thirds of young people who regularly use MP3 players risk early hearing loss because the volume is set too high. It is not simply the fact that headphones bring the sound so close to the ear. There is also the problem that during everyday use people turn up the volume to drown out the background noise of busy streets or public transport.

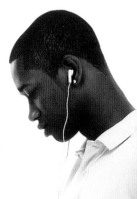

Young people who listen to personal audio devices for more than 7 hours a week have been shown to require louder minimum volumes than the rest of us in order to be able to hear. Yet RNID surveys have found that almost 50 per cent of young people who use MP3 players listen for over an hour a day, with a quarter listening for more than 21 hours a week. And 65 per cent listen to volumes above 85dB – a level that the World Health Organization says can damage hearing if played through earphones for more than an hour at a time.

EFFECTIVE EARPLUGS

Many of the earplugs sold in pharmacies and sports shops are designed to keep water out of the ears when swimming and don't offer much protection against noise. For effective noise protection, look for earplugs specifically designed for the purpose. These have an SNR – simplified noise-level reduction – rating of at least 20dB.

Earplugs designed specially for musicians – and great for clubbers – are called flat attenuators or flat response earplugs. If you use them, the music is just as exciting and you don't lose any of the frequencies – it's just a bit quieter. Those made for professionals are so much smaller than standard earplugs that they are barely noticeable.

PLAY IT TO THE MAX

Alarmingly, 85dB represents roughly the loudness of noise you experience when the volume on your radio or music player is turned up only a quarter of the way towards maximum. When the volume is cranked up to the maximum 120dB, an MP3 user may have less than 15 minutes before suffering some hearing damage. Most users questioned were blissfully unaware that they were putting their hearing at risk – and the RNID is now campaigning to get manufacturers to put warnings on packaging about the dangers of listening to music at levels that are too loud. It also advises users to buy in-ear filters for headphones – these cancel out background noise and produce clear sound at lower, safer volume levels.

worthwhile lifestyle changes

The World Health Organization says that excessive noise exposure is the major avoidable cause of hearing loss. But it is not the only one. There are other influences on your hearing, many of which you, or your GP, can do something about. Surprisingly, lack of exercise and tooth decay are linked to hearing loss. Many medications can affect our hearing or cause tinnitus (see pages 146-147) but often a simple change of prescription can solve the problem. Poor blood circulation to the delicate nerve cells of the inner ear may affect the ear's performance, causing problems with hearing and balance. Therefore, a healthy diet and regular exercise may help to reduce the likelihood of hearing loss. Diabetes or high blood pressure should also be properly monitored and treated.

STOP SMOKING FOR THE SAKE OF YOUR EARS

According to a study of almost 4,000 people in Wisconsin in the USA, people who smoke have almost a 70 per cent higher risk of hearing loss than non-smokers. It seems that smoking reduces oxygen supply to the cochlea, impairing its function. So, if you value your hearing, stop smoking. If you need help, see your GP, or for online advice go to www.quit.org.uk.

top tips for
avoiding noise damage

The more prolonged your exposure to noise and the higher the volume, the greater your chance of hearing loss, but once the exposure ceases no further damage will be done. If you notice hearing loss after exposure to loud noise, it will usually (but not always) improve in the following hours or days. Here are ten ways to limit avoidable noise as much as possible, and safeguard your ears when exposed to unavoidable noise:

- Limit the time that you spend listening to noise for entertainment.
- Reduce volume levels on stereos, TVs and iPods.
- If you use an MP3 or iPod, wear in-ear filters to cancel out background noise.
- Wear proper earplugs or ear defenders whenever you cannot avoid exposure to loud noise, for example when mowing the lawn or using power tools; cotton wool and other homemade plugs are ineffective.
- When in a noisy environment, try to go elsewhere for regular short breaks.
- Distance diminishes the effective decibel level that reaches the ear. Get as far away as possible from unavoidably loud sounds – don't sit or stand next to loudspeakers at a concert, for example.
- If you are provided with ear defenders at work, use them.
- Keep your car windows closed when driving on busy roads.
- Reduce outside traffic and other noise in your home by, for example, installing double glazing, hanging heavy curtains or planting trees or shrubs between you and the road.
- Reduce your stress levels. It is often our emotional response to irritating noise that damages our general health. So, if noise is getting you down, go for a walk somewhere quieter, or soak in a hot bath, or learn to meditate the stress away.

IS THERE A SNORER IN YOUR BED?

You have done everything you can to turn down the volume in your world, so you may feel entitled to a good night's sleep. But if your partner snores, your hearing could be endangered even as you sleep. The noise of snoring can be louder than city traffic. Tape-record your partner if you need to prove your point – and then persuade him or her to see the doctor in case there's a medical solution. If not, you could wear earplugs in bed – ask your chemist about special ones designed to combat low-frequency snoring sounds.

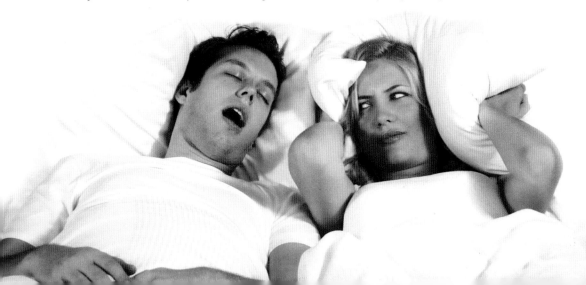

JOG YOUR WAY TO BETTER HEARING

We all know that exercise is beneficial for our general health, but how many people know that it's also good for our hearing? Research has shown that the more physically active we are, the better our hearing is likely to be, because exercise reduces the risk of arterial disease that can damage the inner ear. But a few small studies suggest that taking strenuous exercise at the same time as listening to loud music, especially music relayed through headphones, may increase the likelihood of developing noise-induced hearing loss. It is thought that the physical changes that occur during exercise may make the inner ear more vulnerable to noise damage. So don't listen to loud music on your headphones when you jog – and think about asking your fitness coach to turn down the volume of that upbeat motivational music.

KEEP YOUR TEETH, KEEP YOUR HEARING

It seems that the better the state of your teeth, the less likely you are to lose hearing with age, but it's not clear why. In a study comparing dental health and hearing loss in more than 1,000 people, researchers found that every missing tooth was linked with a doubling in the risk of hearing loss. Also, dental disease has been linked with a raised risk of heart disease, so it could contribute to arterial furring in the ear as well. Whatever the reason for the link between dental and aural health, it's worth looking after your teeth, so pay attention to dental hygiene and have regular check-ups.

feed your ears

In the same way that a healthy lifestyle can bring great benefits to your eyes, it will also do your ears a lot of good. Research studies have shown that, even among people with existing hearing loss, the hearing threshold (the minimum volume at which sound is heard) can improve, and tinnitus (persistent, irritating sound in the ears) can diminish, in those whose diet excludes refined sugars and includes a high proportion of whole raw foods such as vegetables, nuts and seeds.

THE FAT CONNECTION

Chapter 7 drew attention to the Mabaan people of Sudan, who do not appear to be afflicted by age-related hearing loss. One possible reason is that they live a pretty quiet life compared with people in the West. But Dr Samuel Rosen, the New York ear surgeon who originally studied the

Mabaan in 1962, also pointed out that they eat practically no meat or saturated fat. And, in addition to sharp hearing, they have low blood pressure and low cholesterol levels even in their seventies.

To test his hypothesis that this was another factor in keeping sharp hearing into old age, Dr Rosen studied male patients in two long-term residential institutions in Finland, where the intake of cheese, butter and fatty meat is among the highest in the world – as is the incidence of heart disease. He gave the men in one hospital a low-fat diet for five years, while leaving the diet of the men in the other hospital unchanged. As expected, levels of cholesterol and heart disease dropped in men on the low-fat diet – and in

Men aged 50 to 59 in the group following a low-fat diet had better hearing levels than men a decade younger.

addition their hearing improved compared to the men who continued to eat their usual high-fat foods. In fact, men aged 50 to 59 in the group following a low-fat diet had better hearing levels than men a decade younger in the other hospital.

It seems, therefore, that age-related hearing loss could be due to clogging and hardening of the tiny arteries in the ear. In fact, some scientists now believe that atherosclerosis, the process by which cholesterol deposits are laid down in arteries throughout the body, may be as important a cause of hearing loss as it is of heart disease and other so-called 'diseases of civilisation'.

FREE-RADICAL BUSTERS
The advice to reduce your intake of saturated fat in order to preserve your hearing echoes the dietary advice for good vision in chapter 2. Here is another dietary link that may sound familiar. Researchers studying hearing loss are

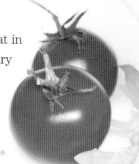

food wisdom for
happy ears

- Cut back on foods high in saturated fats, such as red meats, whole milk, butter, cream and cheese.
- Avoid trans fats and partially hydrogenated vegetable oils, found in margarines, vegetable shortenings, some oils for frying, and many biscuits and other snack foods. They are a major culprit in raising levels of 'bad' fats in the blood and increasing the risk of heart disease.
- Use olive oil for cooking and in salad dressings.
- Limit your intake of processed foods, junk foods, fizzy drinks, sweets, cakes, biscuits and crisps.
- Keep your salt intake to below 6g daily – and don't forget that this includes salt in pre-packed foods, so read the labels.
- Eat more fish, especially oily fish containing omega-3 fatty acids. As well as being good for your eyes, eating oily fish boosts levels of 'good' fats and reduces the risks of cardiovascular disease.
- Eat foods rich in antioxidant vitamins and minerals, especially vegetables, fruit and whole grains.
- Eat small meals regularly – missing meals may lead to overeating.
- Eat grapes and drink grape juice – and wine, in moderation.

Limit your intake of processed foods, junk foods, fizzy drinks, sweets, cakes, biscuits and crisps.

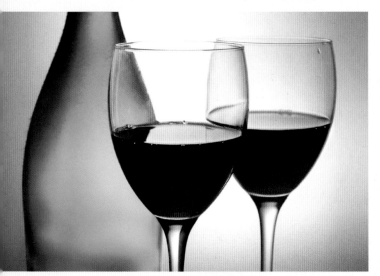

GLORIOUS GRAPES

Grapes, red wine, purple grape juice and peanuts are all good sources of a powerful antioxidant called resveratrol. Some studies suggest that the antioxidant may help to protect against free radical damage to the inner ear, which can result in hearing loss. Resveratrol is known to be good for your heart – and further studies may confirm its hearing benefits. Meanwhile, a well-balanced antioxidant-rich diet will undoubtedly boost your general health.

accumulating evidence to suggest that antioxidant vitamins and minerals may also help to protect your hearing. This is consistent with the studies that have linked exposure to noise with the formation of dangerous free-radical compounds in the ear (see page 124) – because antioxidants effectively mop up free radicals. You can read more about specific studies on vitamin and mineral supplements – and some hearing-friendly herbs – in the rest of this chapter.

supplementary benefits

Vitamins and minerals are vital for all bodily functions. In most cases, a healthy, well-balanced diet will protect against any vitamin and mineral deficiency, but there are times when supplements have a role to play in sustaining health. There are claims by the health-food industry that vitamin and mineral supplements can boost the functions of the body, including eyesight and hearing, but, while they may be valid, not all these claims have been substantiated by vigorous scientific research, so try increasing your intake of appropriate vitamin and mineral-rich foods before taking supplements.

VITAMINS AND MINERALS FROM FOODS

Vitamin D Salmon, herring, sardines, egg yolk and cod liver oil are all sources of vitamin D; it is also made in our skin when we are out in the sun. Vitamin D's importance to hearing is indirect: it is needed to enable our bodies to absorb calcium – and, like other bones in the body, the tiny ossicles in the middle ear need calcium to keep them strong. If you don't get enough vitamin D from your diet or from sunshine – you need about 10 to 20 minutes a day – then supplements could be useful, particularly during the long dark days of winter.

Folate One of the B vitamins, folate, is found in green leafy vegetables, chickpeas and lentils. Low levels of folate have been linked with hearing loss. A Dutch study published in *Annals of Internal Medicine* in January 2007 found that dietary supplementation with folic acid for three years reduced age-related hearing loss in a group of older men and women. But the Netherlands – unlike, say, the USA – does not have a programme of fortifying food with folic acid, so baseline levels in the Dutch population were low initially. More research is needed before the finding can be generalised to include other countries. Since many people are deficient in folate, boosting your dietary intake may be a sensible precaution.

Zinc This mineral is found in high-protein foods including oysters, beef, pork, lamb, peanuts, peanut butter and pulses. A small amount of research has linked low zinc levels to both hearing loss and tinnitus. In some studies, zinc supplementation has been reported to improve symptoms. However, until there is more concrete evidence, it's probably worth eating plenty of zinc-containing foods rather than taking supplements.

Magnesium Foods that provide a good source of this mineral include avocados, nuts and leafy green vegetables such as spinach. Magnesium is an important component of the hair cells in the inner ear. Several

Avocados are a good source of magnesium.

studies have shown that magnesium helps to protect against noise-induced hearing loss in both animals and humans. In one study, teenagers took a magnesium supplement before going to a rock concert. Although it didn't entirely block the damaging effects of noise, there was less change to their hearing thresholds afterwards.

SIMPLE SUPPLEMENTS

Vitamin C One experiment at the University of Buffalo in New York State showed that guinea pigs raised on a diet supplemented with vitamin C gained significant protection against the effects of noise. Those in charge of the study admit that more research in humans is needed, but ask, 'Wouldn't it be great if there was a pill you could take before stepping into a night club, or one that soldiers could take before entering the battlefield?' However, while we might be able to predict exposure to high noise levels at our place of work or at a rock concert, much of our experience of loud noise is sudden and unpredictable. Perhaps, suggest the researchers, we should take daily supplements of vitamin C 'just in case'.

Aspirin and vitamin E More exciting is the idea that antioxidants might be used to treat acute noise-induced hearing loss (NIHL). Scientists studying NIHL have discovered that as well as the release of free radicals immediately following the noise, there is a second peak a few days later. Researchers at the University of Michigan demonstrated that antioxidants (in this case, aspirin and vitamin E) given up to three days after noise exposure still significantly reduced hearing loss in guinea pigs. Hearing damage after exposure to very loud noise has always been thought untreatable; now, for the first time, scientists are suggesting the possibility of a 'window of opportunity' in which at least some damage incurred by noise exposure might be prevented. Further research in humans is needed.

ACE rescue therapy? The same team also found that a combination of high doses of vitamins A, C and E, plus magnesium, taken an hour before noise exposure and continued daily for five days, prevented permanent

Hearing damage after exposure to very loud noise has always been thought untreatable; now, for the first time, scientists are suggesting the possibility of a 'window of opportunity' in which some damage might be prevented.

noise-induced hearing loss in animals exposed to sounds as loud as a jet engine on take-off at close range. They plan to conduct clinical trials of a hearing-protection tablet or snack bar that people could have before going to work in noisy environments or watching motor racing or live bands – perhaps even before turning on their iPods. These micronutrients might even work as a 'morning-after' treatment to minimise hearing damage in soldiers, musicians, pilots, construction workers and others following exposure to potentially dangerous noise levels.

Alpha-lipoic acid While little is known about the effects in humans, animal experiments suggest that, when combined with vitamin E, alpha-lipoic acid, a powerful antioxidant supplement, protects the auditory nerve and can help to counter free radical damage. Good food sources of alpha-lipoic acid include spinach, broccoli, beef, yeast (particularly brewer's yeast) and some offal, such as kidneys and the heart.

Glutathione Another antioxidant that protects the auditory nerve against damage from free radicals is glutathione. Glutathione is also important for brain function, and naturally occurring levels in the body have been shown to decline with age – so glutathione supplements may also benefit your hearing by reducing age-related damage to the hearing centres of your brain. Animal studies at the University of Michigan in the USA and the University of Tokyo in Japan suggest that glutathione may also limit the cochlear damage associated with noise-induced hearing loss, but further research in humans is needed.

HEALING HERBS?

Butcher's broom A herb called butcher's broom, a member of the lily family related to asparagus, is used by herbalists to relieve inflammation and weakness in the veins that impairs circulation, known as venous insufficiency. It has been reported to help alleviate the symptoms of ear infections, but there is little formal research to support this.

Ginkgo biloba An extract of the maidenhair tree, ginkgo biloba is a traditional herbal remedy reputed to boost blood circulation and long used to treat tinnitus (persistent, irritating sound in the ears). Patients with both tinnitus and loss of hearing, which often go together, frequently report that it improves their hearing as well. But, while experiments as long ago as 1975 showed that ginkgo could prevent noise-induced damage to the auditory nerve in animals, a review published in 2004 showed no evidence for the reported benefits of ginkgo in humans.

HOMEOPATHY

Vertigoheel® A combination homoeopathic remedy called Vertigoheel® is used to treat vertigo (dizziness) and related balance disorders that can stem from ear disease. Formal clinical studies in Germany suggested that the remedy reduced the frequency, duration and intensity of vertigo attacks as effectively as the standard drug treatment, betahistine – although some experts question the efficacy of betahistine itself.

your hearing protection plan

You now know what you can do to Protect your hearing. And although the traditional view is that hearing loss with age is inevitable and there is not much that can be done to prevent it, this is not always the case. In fact, this view is increasingly being challenged as researchers understand more about the mechanisms underlying hearing loss and factors that may protect against it. By following the four steps of your *Smart Sense Plan*, you are well on your way to preserving good hearing for life.

The second step of your PACE strategy is to Assess your hearing regularly, so that you can spot any changes quickly and take action. So, as well as protecting your hearing by avoiding excessive noise and adopting a healthy diet and lifestyle, have a hearing test regularly and consult your GP if you develop any symptoms. In the next chapter you will read about conditions that could impair your hearing or cause other symptoms, and what to do about them.

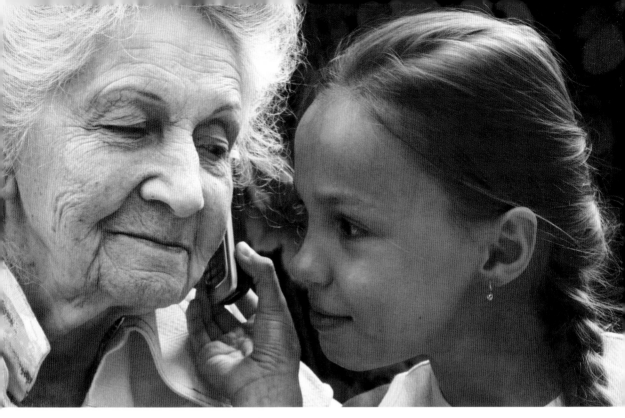

9   What's the problem?

Most people with faulty hearing don't want to admit that there's a problem. All those connotations of doddery great-aunts and ugly plastic hearing aids ... all that wretched business of getting old. Perhaps it's not surprising, then, that some wait for as long as 15 years before seeking help after their hearing begins to fail.

A survey by the RNID confirms that the main reason we don't face up to hearing problems is embarrassment. Many people believe that others will think they are 'past it' or will treat them like idiots if they need to wear a hearing aid. In addition, the survey found that nearly three-quarters of people with impaired hearing who had not seen their doctor or a hearing specialist said that they did not think their hearing was 'bad enough' to warrant getting help. There are many good reasons not to fall into this trap.

So if you answered 'yes' to any of the questions in the test at the start of chapter 7 (see page 117), then have a check-up. If your family complains that you are not hearing them properly, it is probably not because they are

10 reasons why
you should act now

- Many hearing problems are correctable, so, if you don't receive treatment, you are needlessly missing out on many of the joys of hearing, and on being able to communicate properly with your family and others around you.
- Poor hearing may hamper your work, hobbies and social life. Even simple everyday activities, such as making telephone calls or going shopping, can become major sources of frustration. This adds pointless stress to your life.
- In some cases, the degree of hearing loss will worsen with time – possibly irrevocably – when treatment might have prevented this and protected the hearing you've got.
- Even if there isn't a specific treatment, there is often a lot you can do to compensate for hearing loss.
- Hearing loss can be a symptom of other disorders and may alert your GP to something else that requires treatment, so ignoring it could damage your health in other ways.
- Often, hearing loss and associated symptoms such as tinnitus (persistent, irritating sound in the ears) are side effects of medications – so a simple change of drug could alleviate the problem and prevent further damage.
- If a hearing aid is recommended as the best solution, don't despair; modern aids may be more efficient and less noticeable than you think.
- The best time to adjust to a hearing aid and learn how to use it is when your hearing loss is minimal, so if you wait it may be more difficult.
- Hearing loss can be hazardous. If, for example, you can't hear traffic in the streets properly, you're at greater risk of accidents because you may miss the sound of an approaching car or a siren. At home or in a hotel, you could miss smoke or fire alarms or a knock at the door alerting you to danger.
- Hearing loss can lead to social isolation. People who are hard of hearing tend to avoid group conversation and social interaction, and eventually become reclusive.

mumbling – however much you may want to believe otherwise. It is really important to have any problem diagnosed. Your GP can arrange a hearing test and, if necessary, refer you to a specialist. Government guidelines say that no patient should have to wait more than 18 weeks from the time of referral to receiving treatment.

NHS SCREENING AT 55?

More than one in ten middle-aged people in Britain have a moderate to severe hearing problem. This alarming statistic was revealed in November 2007, following a large NHS trial that offered simple 30-second hearing

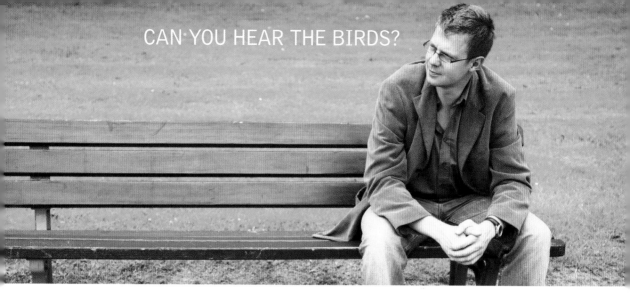

CAN YOU HEAR THE BIRDS?

tests to 35,000 people aged 55 to 74 across Britain. Although only 3 per cent of the sample already had hearing aids, 12 per cent were found to have moderate or severe hearing loss.

Professor Adrian Davis, the director of the Medical Research Council Hearing and Communication Group, who led the study, explained that routine screening for hearing loss is 'incredibly effective' and could offer 'substantial benefits', because, instead of living with hearing difficulties for 10 to 15 years before seeking help, people could vastly enhance their quality of life by acting sooner.

The government is considering the results of the study, with a view to introducing a national programme of routine screening for hearing, possibly by 2013. The RNID supports mass screening and earlier testing. The organisation's spokesperson Emma Harrison observes that the average age for a first hearing test is over 70 – yet, by that age, 60 per cent of people already have a significant hearing loss. 'Widespread screening could improve the quality of life for millions of people,' she says.

CAN YOU HEAR THE BIRDS SINGING?

People frequently assume that hearing loss means simply that the volume of the world is turned down. However, there are many different ways in which hearing loss can be experienced.

Quite often, we lose high-frequency sounds first, making it hard to hear high-pitched voices and sounds such as birdsong, waves and rustling leaves. Certain speech sounds – 's', 'sh', 'ch' and 'f' or 'p', 'k' and 't' – may be difficult to distinguish, so it's more of a challenge than it used to be to understand what people are saying. Some people experience distortion of sounds, fluctuating hearing impairment or even hypersensitivity to certain noises, a phenomenon known as hyperacusis (see page 150). But it's not only your hearing that is affected. Some ear problems disturb the delicate balance mechanisms of the inner ear, leading to balance disorders or dizziness. Many people also experience tinnitus (persistent, irritating sound in the ears, see page 149). And individual ear problems may cause other symptoms such as pain or discharge.

Some experts predict that the number of people living with hearing loss will have almost doubled by 2030.

A GROWING PHENOMENON

In both the UK and the USA, loss of hearing is the third most common chronic condition among older people after arthritis and high blood pressure. And the numbers are expected to rise. The two main reasons for this are that we are living longer and the huge post-war 'baby boomer' generation is now reaching retirement age; a third factor is the large number of younger people who are experiencing noise-induced hearing loss. In fact, some experts predict that the number of people living with hearing loss will have almost doubled by 2030. So stick to your *Smart Sense Plan* to avoid becoming one of them.

types of hearing loss

The two main types of deafness are known medically as conductive and sensorineural hearing loss. The difference depends on what and where the problem is. Some people have mixed hearing loss, in which problems coexist in the outer or middle and the inner ear, leading to combined conductive and sensorineural loss. Other types are congenital hearing loss and central hearing loss.

Conductive hearing loss is caused by anything that blocks the transmission of soundwaves on their passage from the outer to the inner ear – earwax is a common cause. This type of problem may affect one ear or both ears and can often be treated with drugs or an operation. Specific therapies are discussed in chapter 10.

Sensorineural hearing loss, or nerve-related hearing loss, is due to interference with the conversion of soundwaves into an electrical signal in the inner ear, or the transmission of this signal to the brain. This is the most common type of hearing loss among adults, usually affecting both

hearing aid FAQs

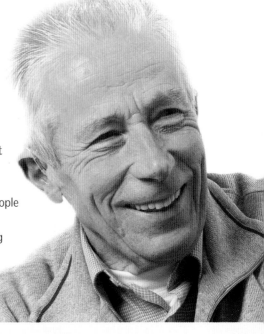

Q 'If I am referred to an NHS specialist, how long will I have to wait?'

A Waiting times are getting shorter. The government's target is that all patients with hearing loss should be seen and treated within 18 weeks of referral. Since age-related deterioration is the commonest cause of hearing loss in people over 60, hearing aids remain the main treatment. For this reason, some older patients are referred directly to hearing specialists or audiologists for hearing-aid assessment. Other older patients and those aged under 60 with hearing loss will be referred to a hospital ear, nose and throat (ENT) specialist.

Q 'Will I be offered a large, ugly hearing aid or do the NHS now supply more discreet ones?'

A The NHS now offers digital aids. These are mainly behind-the-ear devices, though they are more subtle than they used to be. Cosmetic and specialist aids and 'in-canal' aids are not usually available on the NHS.

Q 'What sort of support will I get after my NHS hearing aid has been fitted?'

A Once you are 'in the system' you will receive NHS back-up from the audiology department that supplied the device. They will help you with any fitting or other issues, and supply and fit replacement batteries and parts when necessary. Note that NHS aids remain the property of the NHS.

Q 'If I don't want to wait, can I be referred to a private specialist?'

A Your GP can refer you for private ENT assessment or can recommend a private hearing aid supplier. Alternatively, you can get help from the Hearing Aid Council – go to http://thehearingaidcouncil.org.uk/ or telephone 020 3102 4030, or try www.bshaa.com – the website of the British Society of Hearing Aid Audiologists.

Q 'If a friend recommends a good private specialist, do I need a referral or can I just make an appointment?'

A You don't need a referral; you can simply phone for an appointment.

Q 'How much will a state-of-the-art hearing aid cost?'

A You can pay anything from £300 to £3,000 privately, depending on what you choose. The cheaper private aids are generally not as sophisticated as the standard NHS aid.

Q 'What about those adverts for tiny, but costly, "miracle" hearing aids?'

A Be cautious. You can't always believe advertisements, nor be sure that the supplier will give you an unbiased opinion about whether the device is right for you. Choose a supplier by personal recommendation and ask about refunds – good suppliers will generally give a total or partial refund if you are not happy after four weeks.

ears and sometimes accompanied by tinnitus. Sound intensity and quality may both be impaired. The commonest complaint is difficulty in hearing or interpreting speech, especially against background noise. Some problems can be solved before permanent damage occurs. If a medication is the cause, for example, irreversible hearing loss may be avoided if it is stopped in time. A hearing aid, which amplifies sound to increase the intensity of the signal reaching the inner ear, can help most of those people affected.

Congenital hearing loss is present from birth. This type of hearing loss may be conductive, sensorineural or both. It may be caused by an inherited disorder or by the presence of an infection – when, for example, a pregnant woman contracts German measles (rubella), which then affects her developing baby. Alternatively, congenital hearing loss can happen as a result of an injury to the baby sustained during birth.

Central hearing loss is a rare condition that is caused by damage or impairment to the auditory pathways or centres in the brain. Possible causes of central hearing loss include multiple sclerosis, brain tumours and strokes.

bangs and blockages
CAUSES OF CONDUCTIVE HEARING LOSS

Perforated eardrum Sometimes, head injury or other accidental trauma damages the structures of the outer or middle ear. Most common is a perforated eardrum, where the delicate membrane dividing the outer from the middle ear is damaged. This can happen as a result of a blow to the ear, rapid pressure changes when flying or scuba diving, the pressure blast of an explosion or other very loud noise, a build-up of fluid pressure due to untreated middle ear infection or, most commonly, misguided attempts to poke around in the ear canal to clear out wax. A perforated eardrum may

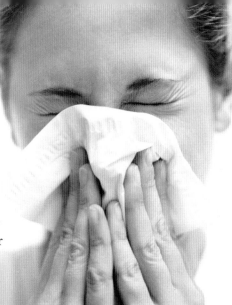

cause short-term pain, temporarily reduced hearing and sometimes a discharge, but it usually heals on its own within a few weeks. In the meantime, keep your ear dry – water from showering or swimming could lead to infection and permanent damage.

Blocked ear A build-up of wax or a foreign body lodged in the ear canal dulls your hearing because the sound waves can't reach the eardrum. Wax is there for a reason – it's sticky, to trap dirt, dust and germs, and contains lysozyme, the natural antibacterial substance

Ordinary coughs and colds can lead to fluid build-up and swelling or blockage of the Eustachian tubes, causing muffled hearing and sometimes tinnitus.

present in tears. But sometimes you can end up with a lump of wax that interferes with hearing. Never push cotton buds deep into your ear– not only could you damage the eardrum but you may also push the wax further down and compact it against the drum. Your practice nurse can check your ears for wax and clean them if need be.

Colds, flu and allergies Ordinary coughs and colds, flu, tonsillitis and sinusitis can lead to fluid build-up and swelling or blockage of the Eustachian tubes, causing muffled hearing and sometimes tinnitus. There may also be earache and a raised temperature. Allergies and enlarged adenoids can have a similar effect. When fluid builds up in the middle ear and gets infected, it's known as otitis media – a common complaint in young children because their Eustachian tubes are very short and horizontal.

think SENSE ● ● ●

TWO HOME REMEDIES

● If you're prone to excess wax, stop the problem by using a drop or two of warmed olive oil in your ear and leaving overnight – plugged with a bung of cotton wool, and place a towel under your head to protect your pillows. A weekly treatment should keep wax under control.

● For really stubborn wax, try this alternative: buy a bottle of 3 per cent hydrogen peroxide and a dropper bottle from the chemist. Put about a tablespoon in half a cup of warm water and use the dropper to place a few drops in your ear – tilt your head sideways over a sink to do this. Don't worry if you hear bubbling – it's just the peroxide working on the wax. Wait until the bubbling stops, then tilt your head the other way over an old towel to let what's in your ear out. Then repeat with the other ear. **Warning** Don't stick the end of the dropper into the ear, and don't do this if you have any other ear problems, such as pain, infection or a burst drum. You may have to repeat the procedure several times to get the wax out.

Continued on p148 ➤

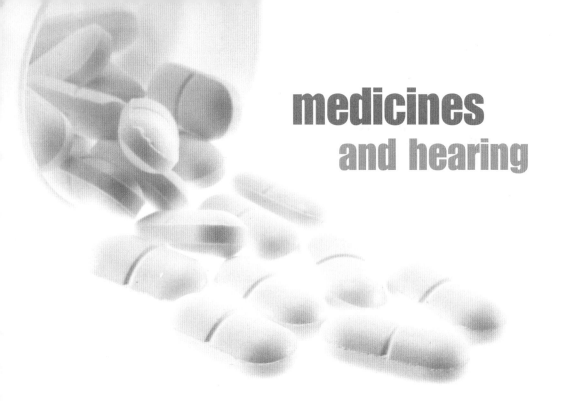

medicines
and hearing

Many prescribed or over-the-counter medications can cause hearing loss, tinnitus or both. These are called 'ototoxic', meaning toxic to the ear. They may damage the hair cells of the inner ear or interfere with the auditory nerve that transmits hearing signals to the brain.

In addition, some drugs distort sounds and interfere with the quality and clarity of hearing, or disturb the delicate mechanisms of the inner ear, causing balance problems and dizziness. Vapours and solvents such as cleaning fluids or petrol can have similar effects, as can some industrial chemicals and environmental pollutants. Heavy metal poisoning – such as with lead or mercury – can lead to hearing loss or balance problems.

Ototoxic symptoms are frequently temporary and clear up if the medication is stopped quickly enough – so tell your GP immediately about any symptoms. Aspirin, if it is taken in high doses, can trigger tinnitus, but this will disappear once you stop taking it.

ASSESSING THE RISK

There are hundreds of drugs that may have ototoxic side effects, but bear in mind that some people are more genetically susceptible to certain drugs than others. In many instances, especially in the case of anti-cancer drugs, the benefits of taking the medication clearly outweigh the dangers. Other examples pose a risk only when taken in high doses. Aspirin, for example, is an important drug in the prevention of heart attacks and is not ototoxic when taken at the doses recommended for heart protection.

EAR ADVERSARIES

Among the medications that may be ototoxic, the main culprits are:

- High-dose aspirin.
- High-dose NSAIDs (non-steroidal anti-inflammatory drugs) such as ibuprofen and indomethacin.
- Many antibiotics, especially aminoglycosides such as gentamicin, streptomycin and neomycin, especially when they are injected into the blood or into the ear.
- Anti-malarial drugs containing quinine.
- Diuretics such as frusemide (Lasix) in high doses.
- Heart and blood-pressure medications, such as calcium-channel blockers (rare).
- Hormones, such as oral contraceptives and hormone replacement therapies (in patients with otosclerosis, see page 148).
- Some anti-cancer (cytotoxic) drugs (though these may well be essential medicines).

DON'T LET DRUGS DAMAGE YOUR EARS

While ototoxic reactions are relatively rare for most drugs, it is a good idea to minimise the risk of a medication affecting your hearing. Here are some guidelines:

- Before you take any drug, ask your pharmacist or check the label or package insert to see whether ear symptoms are listed among the side effects.
- If your family has a history of ear problems, or you've reacted to drugs before, tell your GP.
- Tell your doctor if you've had or have any hearing problems, tinnitus, balance problems or dizziness.
- Avoid very noisy places while you are taking the medication; damage from the noise could add to that of the drug.
- Never take more than the recommended dose.
- While taking any drug, and for a week or two afterwards, watch for any odd symptoms, however slight, and report them to your GP at once. Early signals of a reaction include dizziness, tinnitus, a fullness or pressure in your ears, worsening of existing hearing loss or tinnitus, and vertigo (see page 150).

Cysts In rare instances, repeated ear infections can lead to collapse of the eardrum, forming a retraction pocket in the middle ear. Trapped skin cells may become infected and create a cyst (cholesteatoma).Left untreated, the cyst can grow and damage the middle ear structures, causing hearing loss and dizziness. Other symptoms include a sensation of fullness in one ear, a smelly discharge, night-time earache in or behind the ear, and even muscle weakness on the side of the face closest to that ear.

Otosclerosis This rare condition causes conductive hearing loss. As a result of abnormal bone growth, one (or more) of the ossicles in the middle ear becomes less mobile, so it cannot transmit sound vibrations properly. Otosclerosis can also cause dizziness, balance disorders and tinnitus. The condition often runs in families and affects more females than males. The hearing loss often becomes apparent during and following pregnancy.

nerve messages interrupted
CAUSES OF SENSORINEURAL HEARING LOSS

Acoustic trauma A sudden burst of intense noise, such as a gunshot, can cause transient deafness by damaging the hair cells in the cochlea. In severe cases, this 'acoustic trauma' can lead to permanent deafness.

Age-related hearing loss The most common hearing diagnosis is age-related hearing loss, known medically as presbyacusis. Here are some of the underlying factors that are thought to be linked to the problem:

- Genes Some people seem more likely to develop hearing impairment with age than others. This could be an inherited genetic weakness or they may be more vulnerable to other sources of hearing damage.
- Atherosclerosis Clogged and narrowed arteries in the body mean that less blood and oxygen reach the cochlea; the resulting increase in free-radical formation damages hair cells responsible for sound detection.
- Poor diet, lack of exercise, obesity Over-eating, eating too much saturated fat or sugar, or too many junk foods causes obesity, which is linked to atherosclerosis. Lack of exercise exacerbates the problem.
- Diabetes Atherosclerosis is accelerated in people with diabetes, who also have other vascular changes that may cut blood flow to the cochlea.
- Noise Long-term exposure to noisy environments is thought to lead to an accumulation of inner-ear damage and eventual hearing loss.
- Drugs and toxins Many drugs can damage our hearing and the chance of this increases the older we get and the more medications we are prescribed. Exposure to toxins can cause similar harm.

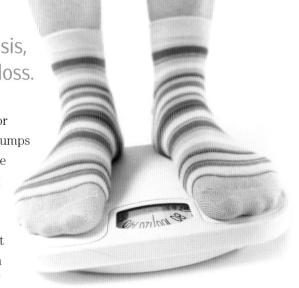

Obesity is linked to atherosclerosis, which can cause hearing loss.

Head injury or infection If a head injury, or surgery, or an infection such as meningitis, mumps or measles affects the inner ear, it can damage the hair cells or the auditory nerve conveying sound information to the brain, sometimes leading to permanent hearing impairment.

Ménière's disease This condition can affect one or both ears. Its main symptom is sudden attacks of severe vertigo – a horrible sense of spinning and loss of balance. There may also be tinnitus, hearing loss and a feeling of pressure in the ear. Sometimes the condition runs in families, and it seems to be more common in people who suffer from migraine. Although the cause of Ménière's disease is not directly related to excessive salt intake, a drastic cut in salt from the diet may help symptoms to subside in some sufferers.

Benign tumour Sometimes a non-cancerous tumour known as an acoustic neuroma grows on the auditory nerve conveying sound signals to the brain. This leads to hearing loss, together with tinnitus, headaches, dizziness and numb feelings in the face. Such a tumour can remain small, and its size can be monitored by regular scanning. It can be treated by surgery or radiotherapy if it is showing signs of enlargement.

tinnitus – sound in the ears

The term 'tinnitus' comes from a Latin word meaning 'ringing'. While the condition is frequently described as a ringing in the head, some people perceive a sound more like a high-pitched whine; others hear a hiss, a buzz, a hum or a loud whistle like that from an old-fashioned whistling kettle. Or you might hear a roaring, like waves on a pebbly shore, or perhaps a clicking sound.

Almost any ear condition can cause tinnitus. If you experience such noises occasionally and for just a minute or two, don't panic – noises in the ear can arise if you are stressed or tired. But if you get persistent tinnitus, either on its own or with hearing loss, then seek medical help fast. The noise may be high or low-pitched, constant or come in waves or pulses, and may occur on one or both sides, or be experienced in your head.

Tinnitus can be an important clue to ear disease and possible hearing damage, including from noise or drugs. It sometimes occurs in association with general health problems such as cardiovascular disease, anaemia or an under-active thyroid. It is estimated to affect up to one in ten people in the UK, and can cause difficulty concentrating, sleep disturbance, forgetfulness, frustration and sometimes depression. Fortunately there's plenty you can do to improve matters, as you'll read in the next chapter.

vertigo – a moving world

Any condition affecting the balance centres in either the ear or the brain may cause vertigo, an unpleasant form of dizziness that makes you feel as if either you or your environment is moving, even when you are still. Those affected can also feel light-headed and unstable. Like seasickness, vertigo may produce nausea and vomiting.

It is estimated that about one in 20 of us has suffered from vertigo or other types of dizziness at some time in our lives, with the figures leaping to one in three people aged over 60 and two in three of those over 80.

Vertigo is normally an inner-ear disorder. It can be caused by a viral infection, a head injury or the side effects of some medications. It can also occur in cardiovascular, neurological or other disorders. Always report any dizziness to your GP in case your medication needs to be reviewed or other causes investigated.

hyperacusis – an intolerable racket

Extreme sensitivity to sound, known as hyperacusis, can make everyday activities very difficult, especially in our noise-filled world. It is thought to affect more than one in 50 adults in the UK. Sometimes experienced separately from other disorders, the condition more often develops along with hearing loss, and is usually accompanied by tinnitus – around 40 per cent of people with tinnitus have hyperacusis, as well. It can also result in earache and a feeling of fullness or pressure in the ears.

The cause of hyperacusis is unknown. It may be a reaction to a medication or follow exposure to a sudden very loud noise, a head injury, surgery or infections. It can also occur with migraine or epilepsy. High-frequency sounds are most often involved – a baby crying or the squealing

Living with tinnitus

Jean Lakins

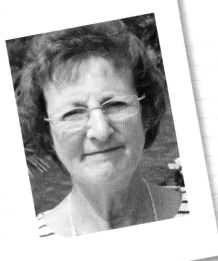

Jean Lakins, a retired community midwife from Broadstone, Dorset, developed tinnitus in 1979 after a prolonged course of antibiotics for a pelvic infection, and started to hear noises in both ears and down the middle of her head 'that just got louder and louder', she says.

'The main sound is like the hissing noise you get from a television set when it's not tuned into a programme.' She became deaf in one ear after an operation in 1994 to remove a cholesteatoma (an abnormal skin growth behind the ear drum) and it was then that the tinnitus became more pronounced. When the ear problem recurred about 11 years ago, it became louder still.

> 'The main sound is like the hissing noise you get from a television set when it's not tuned into a programme.'

Triggers Jean has found that being tired or stressed exacerbates her tinnitus, as does eating chocolate and drinking wine – especially when combined with going to bed late in the evening. 'A good night's sleep helps – but I can't usually get more than about 6 hours as the noise wakes me up,' she says ruefully.

Brain training Jean has several strategies to help her to live with tinnitus. 'You have to learn to keep calm and know how to relax,' she says. Sometimes, this means simply sitting quietly and taking a few deep breaths. It also helps to concentrate on something else: 'I tend to keep a radio on in the house. You can train your brain to listen to something other than the tinnitus.'

Moving forward Jean has spent a couple of years learning sign language as a precaution, just in case she loses the hearing in her other ear. She takes a great deal of care to protect her good ear, and uses earplugs whenever she goes anywhere that's likely to be noisy. She is a voluntary counsellor for her local tinnitus support group, and recommends that anyone with tinnitus get in touch with the British Tinnitus Association (www.tinnitus.org.uk) for information and to find details of their nearest voluntary support counsellor; there are local support groups all over the country. Her mantra is simple: 'Keep healthy, active and occupied, but above all try to live life as normally as possible.'

of brakes can be almost unbearable. But sometimes everyday sounds – running water from a tap or the rustle as newspaper pages are turned – may be experienced as excruciatingly loud. And of course, if people raise their voices to try to overcome any associated hearing loss, the effect is even worse. Devices that can help most affected people to re-train their hearing are discussed in chapter 10.

recruitment – 'no need to shout ...'

The main feature of 'recruitment' is that sounds get too loud too quickly. Recruitment is always a symptom of hearing loss where some of the hair cells in the cochlea have died off. To compensate for the loss of signals at certain frequencies, the brain tries to recruit adjacent cells to do the job. These cells then send a double signal, both for their own and the missing frequency, making certain sounds seem twice as loud as normal. If the loss of hair cells is severe, the recruited cells may even operate for many missing ones at once – making the perceived sound louder still.

You may not be able to hear a sound at all until the recruited cells start working, then, when you can, the volume is multiplied so that the noise is unbearably loud. In such cases, a person suffering from the condition might ask someone to speak up, and then protest, 'No need to shout. I'm not deaf!' Since cells detecting different frequencies are signalling at the same time, the extra-loud sounds are also fuzzy, so people affected may find it hard to distinguish similar-sounding words or they may even experience all speech as meaningless noise.

moving on to correct hearing

If you have any kind of hearing problem, you should now be more aware of it and able to discuss any symptoms that concern you. You have begun to Assess your hearing which, after doing everything you can to Protect it, is the next important step in the PACE strategy that makes up your *Smart Sense Plan*. Make an appointment to see your GP – the sooner you move on to the Correct stage of your plan, the more likely it is that you will be able to retain and even improve the quality of hearing that you have.

The next chapter discusses what can be done to treat ear problems, and looks at the remarkable range of technological equipment that is available to help people with hearing difficulties.

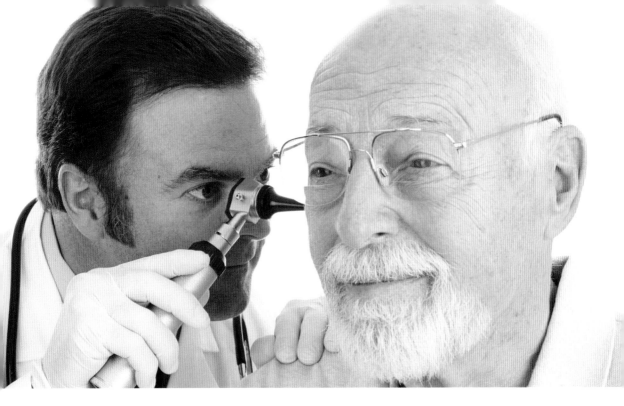

Technology to the rescue

10

So, what can be done to Correct hearing problems? Knowing your options and discovering the best and most appropriate treatment is the next vital part of your Smart Sense Plan. In these pages you'll find out how the experts assess your hearing, and the huge range of treatments, gadgets and help available to enable you to continue to enjoy this precious sense.

Your first port of call should be your GP. He or she will ask you to describe your symptoms and might ask you about any relevant factors in your medical history. For example, have you suffered any head injury or undergone ear surgery? Have you experienced any diseases linked with hearing loss, such as multiple sclerosis, stroke or cardiovascular disease? What medications – prescription or over-the-counter – are you taking? Are you exposed to loud or continuous noise either at work or through hobbies,

Who's who in hearing

You will probably see one of the following specialists, depending on the likely cause of the problem:

- **Audiologist** – someone qualified to identify and assess hearing loss, balance disorders and tinnitus. An audiologist may recommend appropriate treatment, such as a hearing aid, or advise on communication strategies or balance retraining exercises. Audiologists usually work in the audiology clinic of your local hospital or health centre.
- **Audiovestibular physician** – a doctor specialising in audiovestibular medicine: the investigation, diagnosis and non-surgical management of hearing and balance disorders, including tinnitus. Some specialise further in the management of speech and language disorders in children – known as phoniatrics.
- **Ear, nose and throat (ENT) specialist**, also called an otolaryngologist or otorhinolaryngologist – a medical doctor with specialised training in the surgical and medical treatment of conditions of the ears, nose and throat, and also the head and neck. The specialist can diagnose and treat hearing loss, tinnitus, ear infections and balance disorders.

such as shooting? And is there any family history of deafness? Depending on your symptoms, the doctor may look in your ears with a device called an otoscope or auroscope.

Often, if there is a simple, treatable cause for your hearing problem, the doctor might deal with it on the spot – removing earwax, for example, or stopping or changing a medication that could be causing your symptoms. If your doctor suspects an underlying problem, then you may be given further tests or referred to a consultant.

checking your hearing

If your hearing loss can't be rectified by a simple change in prescription or by clearing a wax blockage, don't despair. There's a huge amount that can be done to improve your hearing and make day-to-day life much easier. First, your doctor or audiologist will assess your hearing level, using one or more of the following tests; the first two can be performed in a GP surgery.

WHISPERED VOICE TEST

In this simple screening test, the tester stands at arm's length (about 60cm/2ft) behind you – so you can't lip read – and whispers words or numbers which you are asked to repeat. Each ear is tested separately, while you block the other one with your fingertip. If you can't hear a whisper the tester may gradually increase the volume of speech. This is not a particularly accurate measure but, as a rough guide, the volume of speech needed to hear equates to these degrees of hearing loss:

Quiet whisper:	normal hearing	
Loud whisper:	hearing loss	20-30dB
Quiet voice:	hearing loss	30-45dB
Loud voice:	hearing loss	45-60dB
Shout:	hearing loss	60-80dB

TUNING FORK TESTS

Tuning forks are a simple way to make an initial assessment of hearing loss at different frequencies and to distinguish between conductive and sensorineural (nerve-related) hearing loss (see page 142). The examiner strikes the fork – a metal handle with a small flat plate at one end and two mental prongs at the other – against the edge of a table to make the prongs vibrate, and then holds the flat plate in different places against your head. This does not hurt.

There are two basic tests. Both rely on the fact that the inner ear is normally twice as sensitive to sound waves transmitted through the air as to sound vibrations conducted through skull bone. But someone with conductive hearing loss – where something blocks transmission of soundwaves from the outer to the inner ear – will be less able to hear environmental noise in the affected ear, and so will be more sensitive to skull bone-conducted sound.

● In Weber's test the vibrating fork is placed in the middle of your forehead. If you have normal hearing, you should hear the bone-conducted sound in the middle, or equally in both ears. If you have hearing loss in both ears, the sound may be muted or you may not hear it at all. When there is loss in only one ear, if you hear the sound louder in the affected ear, this suggests conductive hearing loss; if it sounds louder in the better ear this suggests nerve-related hearing loss.

● In Rinne's test, the vibrating fork is first held on one side against the bony lump just behind your ear, called the mastoid process, and then moved about 8cm (3in) away from the ear. You will be asked which sounds louder. If you have normal hearing, the sound will be louder when the fork is held in front of your ear and the sound waves are being conducted through air. If you have conductive hearing loss, you will hear the sound louder when the fork is pressed against the mastoid process and the sound waves are conducted through bone. Confusingly, if you cannot hear at all on one side, you will still experience the bone conduction as louder as the vibrations are transmitted around the skull and heard in the other ear.

PURE-TONE AUDIOMETRY

The most accurate means of assessing any hearing loss is the pure-tone audiogram. It involves the use of an electronic device called an audiometer that produces sounds of different volumes and pitch to identify your hearing threshold – the lowest intensity at which you can hear particular sounds. You are usually asked to sit in a soundproof room or booth wearing headphones and to indicate by pushing a button when you can hear a series of sounds. 'Normal' hearing is detecting most frequencies at 20dB or less. The results are plotted on a chart called an audiogram and can also determine the type of hearing loss – conductive, sensorineural or mixed.

OTHER TESTS

If your hearing loss is suspected to be sensorineural in origin (due to a signalling problem in the inner ear or auditory nerve), you may be advised to have an otoacoustic emission test. This measures the responses of your cochlea to sounds produced by a probe resting in your ear canal, in order to assess how well the hair cells in your inner ear are functioning. You don't have to do anything, and it doesn't hurt.

There's a huge amount that can be done to improve hearing and make day-to-day life much easier.

Another test measures your auditory brainstem response – how the hearing centres in your brain react to sounds. A series of clicks or pips are transmitted through headphones or an earpiece placed in your outer ear canal while you wear electrodes on your scalp and earlobes to detect brainwaves that occur in response. Again, this is painless and you don't need to do anything – the test can even be done on someone asleep or in a coma. It's used to check babies with suspected hearing problems, those who find audiometry difficult to perform, and sometimes for adults with head injuries or to distinguish other types of sensorineural hearing loss.

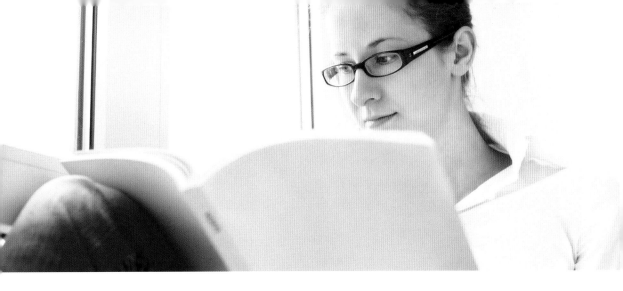

understanding the results

Hearing loss is measured in decibels (dB) relative to normal hearing, on a scale that ranges from 0 to 100. A normal hearing score for an adult is 0 to 20dB; for children it's 0 to 15dB. The higher your score, the higher volumes you need to hear and the worse your hearing – so 100dB hearing loss means virtually complete deafness for that particular frequency.

Mild hearing loss People with mild hearing loss (21-40dB) cannot hear whispers. They may find it difficult to understand speech if there is a lot of background noise, and may also have problems with quiet sounds and certain consonants, especially the soft sibilants, such as f, s and th. They may use lip reading and other facial and gesture cues to help them to hold a conversation. A hearing aid can make a significant difference.

Moderate hearing loss Those with moderate hearing loss (41-65dB) can't hear conversational speech properly and are likely to miss a lot of speech sounds unless they lip read. A hearing aid will help with speech; other gadgets, such as an amplified phone, can resolve everyday obstacles.

Severe hearing loss People with severe hearing loss (66-90dB) cannot hear shouting. They may find it hard to understand speech even with a hearing aid, and may not hear sounds, such as traffic noise. They are likely to rely heavily on lip reading and may use sign language to communicate.

Profound hearing loss People with profound hearing loss (more than 90dB) can't hear even very loud sounds that might be painful for a hearing person – such as aircraft noise at close range. They must rely on lip reading and sign language as hearing aids don't help much. They are unlikely to be able to use a phone, even with amplification, so would benefit from having a textphone. But for some deaf people, a remarkable piece of technology called a cochlear implant (see page 169) can bring vital hearing and communication abilities.

how your GP can help

For simple medical problems that affect your hearing, a GP can often provide effective treatment. A GP or practice nurse can clear your ears of wax or prescribe decongestant or anti-allergy drugs if necessary.

If your hearing loss or tinnitus has begun only recently, your GP will probably check what medicines you are taking – drugs that can damage your hearing (ototoxic) are discussed on pages 144-145. It's also important to tell your doctor about any over-the-counter remedies you use. Although ototoxic drugs affect your inner ear, symptoms usually clear up pretty quickly without damaging the hair cells once you stop taking the medication.

EAR INFECTIONS

In young children, ear infections are common, but most clear up within a few days without any specific treatment. Your GP may prescribe antibiotics for a bacterial infection of the middle ear (otitis media) or for sinusitis. But antibiotics are ineffective against viral infections – and your doctor can't always tell the difference. If your GP decides against antibiotics, he or she might advise you to take decongestants, and will probably suggest that you take painkillers for earache. Your hearing may be muffled for a week or so after an ear infection until any mucus left in the middle ear clears up. If you suffer from recurrent ear infections, fluid build-up or other complications, you may be referred to an ear, nose and throat (ENT) specialist (see page 154).

PERFORATED EARDRUM

As long as you take great care to keep water out of the ear canal – which can cause infection – a perforated eardrum will usually heal within six to eight weeks. If fluid build-up behind the drum due to an infection has

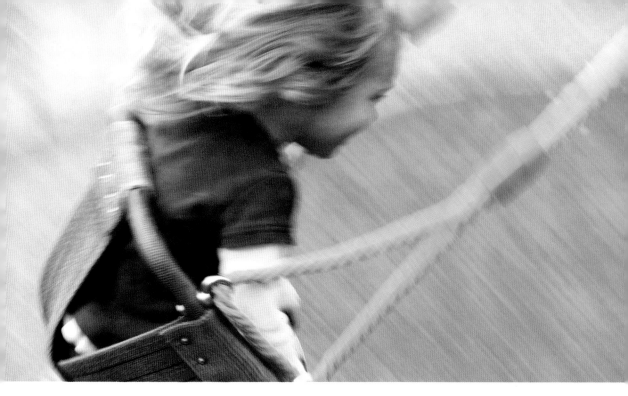

For children, at least, many family doctors take a 'watch and wait' approach, giving antibiotics only if symptoms do not improve within 72 hours.

caused the perforation, your GP may prescribe antibiotics, and will usually ask you to return for check-ups to ensure the hole heals. If it doesn't, or if you have a large perforation, you may be referred for surgery to patch the drum (see page 162).

MÉNIÈRE'S DISEASE

If your doctor suspects Ménière's disease (see page 149), you will probably be referred for further tests, such as a head scan. The cause of Ménière's disease is still not fully understood, but as mentioned in the last chapter, symptoms of the disease are thought to be due to a build-up of fluid in the inner ear. For this reason, some doctors may suggest that you follow a diet that is very low in salt, or they may prescribe a diuretic to reduce fluid retention, although the overall effectiveness of the treatments is still unclear.

If, for any reason, the combination of diet and drugs is not completely successful, you might be referred to an ENT surgeon to consider a variety of surgical options to help to control the attacks of vertigo. In addition, during periods of remission, any residual imbalance may be helped by a balance retraining physiotherapist.

symptom relief

Some ear conditions can't be cured. But there's a great deal that can be done to improve matters, whether you are living with the constant noise of tinnitus, the sudden and painful volume increases of hyperacusis or the dizziness of vertigo.

MAKING TINNITUS EASIER TO LIVE WITH

Tinnitus is stressful – and stress can make it worse – so for some people, sedatives, tranquillisers or antidepressants can be helpful. For others, cognitive behaviour therapy (CBT) works miracles, helping them to change their response and focus away from the noise. Specialists may also recommend listening to music as a distraction, especially at bedtime. If you have impaired hearing, a hearing aid can relieve tinnitus symptoms because louder and clearer external sounds override the internal noises.

White noise A tinnitus masking gadget called a white noise generator produces a soothing, low level sound like a 'shhh', which you set at a level just below or at the same pitch as your tinnitus. If you listen to it regularly, your brain becomes accustomed to the sound and your tinnitus becomes less noticeable. A slightly richer version called pink noise works better for some people.

You can buy white noise CDs, tapes or MP3 downloads for use with ordinary speakers or headphones, or with special pillow speakers at night. Some white noise machines offer a choice of soothing sounds, such as light rain, a waterfall, a bubbling stream or birdsong. The NHS can provide an in-ear device, a bit like a hearing aid, that generates white noise. If you need a hearing aid anyway, there are combination units that do both – ask your audiologist what's available.

Eighty per cent of sufferers find that tinnitus retraining therapy – a combination of white noise and CBT – reduces symptoms dramatically, but you need to persevere: it can take a year or more to achieve full results.

cuttingEDGE

BRAZILIAN BREAKTHROUGH?

Researchers at a hospital in Rio De Janeiro gave acamprosate (Campral) – a drug normally used to treat alcoholism – to 25 tinnitus patients for three months, then compared them with another 25 patients who had received a placebo. Nearly half of those who had taken acamprosate reported more than 50 per cent relief from their symptoms, while more than three quarters had some relief; three said that their tinnitus had disappeared altogether. Scientists speculate that the drug may reduce the excess nerve cell activity underlying the sensation of tinnitus, or it could simply reduce people's awareness of tinnitus. More studies are needed and Action for Tinnitus Research is campaigning to raise funds to pay for the research.

THERAPIES FOR HYPERACUSIS

If you have this uncommon condition, you will probably be referred to an ENT or audiology specialist. A hearing test and perhaps a loudness discomfort test, will gauge the severity of your symptoms. If any underlying cause is identified you may be offered treatment; otherwise hyperacusis retraining therapy – auditory desensitisation and CBT – is the normal course of action.

Pink noise As with tinnitus, noise generators have proved a boon for many people with hyperacusis. 'Pink' noise seems to work better with hyperacusis

Some ear conditions can't be cured. But there's a great deal that can be done to improve matters.

than white noise, because the richer sounds help the ears to become desensitised to the loud sounds of hyperacusis. The treatment involves playing a CD or using an in-ear device to generate pink or white noise at just audible levels, for gradually increasing periods building up to 8 hours a day. This is thought to re-establish tolerance to sound, and while it may take a year or more to work, it appears that perseverance is rewarded, as 90 per cent of people have reported a 'substantial improvement'.

STEADYING A SPINNING WORLD

Vertigo may be triggered by a treatable disorder, such as an ear infection; once the infection clears, the vertigo disappears. But sometimes symptoms are due to a problem known medically as benign paroxysmal positional vertigo (BPPV). This harmless, but infuriating condition causes short episodes of intense dizziness when you move your head in particular directions, especially when rolling over or getting out of bed.

BPPV is thought to be due to debris formed when some of the tiny granules in the vestibular system of the inner ear, that help to detect head movements and gravity, are displaced. These granules float off in the inner ear fluid, irritating movement detectors in the semi-circular canals. You might be able to prevent dizziness simply by avoiding movements that trigger it. Or a doctor or physiotherapist can perform the Epley manoeuvre – manipulating your head with a series of movements that 'clears away' the debris and allows it to settle elsewhere in the inner ear, where it causes no problems. This is simple and often highly successful. Anti-nausea drugs may help to relieve symptoms but no medication cures the condition. BPPV often resolves itself within a few weeks, but can recur.

For other types of vertigo, you may be referred for vestibular rehabilitation therapy (VRT). You will be taught a set of exercises to perform daily, involving progressively more difficult head, eye and walking movements. These are designed to encourage the brain to adapt to the stimuli that provoke vertigo and compensate, irrespective of the cause. They can help to reduce dizziness, improve balance and prevent falls.

surgical solutions

PERFORATED EARDRUM

If you have an eardrum perforation that does not heal, you may be advised to have an operation to repair it, called a tympanoplasty or myringoplasty. It is performed under general anaesthetic either as a day procedure or with an overnight stay in hospital. A tiny piece of tissue is removed from just above your ear to use as a graft. The surgeon then uses a special microscope and minute instruments to lift the eardrum and insert the graft beneath it to close the hole. You have to keep the ear covered with an antibiotic dressing for about three weeks, while the graft heals.

GLUE EAR

In severe cases of otitis media (see Colds, flu and allergies, page 145), surgery can be used to create a hole in the eardrum to allow fluid to drain out. In some cases, especially in children who have persistent fluid accumulation behind the eardrum, the surgeon can insert grommets – tiny plastic tubes that keep a drainage channel open through a hole in the eardrum (see above, right). If enlarged adenoids seem to be provoking repeated infections, these may be surgically removed at the same time.

OTOSCLEROSIS

If your hearing is impaired because of otosclerosis when, as a result of abnormal bone growth, one or more ossicles in the middle ear cannot transmit sound vibrations properly (see page 148), you might be offered surgery. In a delicate operation, which can be performed through the ear

HOW A GROMMET WORKS

The grommet, positioned within the eardrum membrane, creates a hole that allows air to circulate within the middle ear, and fluid in the middle ear to escape or dry out. Short-term grommets are expelled naturally and painlessly by the ear over a period of between 6-15 months, allowing time for the condition to be resolved. In some cases, long-term grommets are inserted and surgically removed after two or three years.

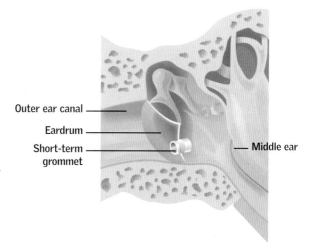

Outer ear canal

Eardrum

Short-term grommet

Middle ear

... the surgeon can insert grommets – tiny plastic tubes that keep the drainage channel open ...

canal, the diseased ossicle is removed and replaced with an artificial ceramic or titanium one. This may also be carried out if the ossicles are damaged by injury or infection. It is usually successful in restoring hearing.

BENIGN TUMOUR

If your doctor suspects a benign tumour, known as acoustic neuroma (see page 149), you will be referred to a specialist and may have a brain scan, to reveal any growth on your auditory nerve. Such tumours usually grow slowly and are non-cancerous, so there's often no need to rush into surgery. If you have hearing loss, tinnitus or balance problems, or if there is concern about the appearance or size of the growth, treatment may be recommended. In some cases radiotherapy may shrink the tumour to manageable proportions; in others, it may require surgical removal. It depends on the size and location of the tumour and on your general health. When small tumours are removed, hearing can often be preserved.

CYSTS

One reason an ear specialist will operate on a perforated eardrum is to reduce the chance of a cystic infection called a cholesteatoma, which can also occur after middle ear infections (see page 145). The cysts are initially treated with careful ear cleaning and antibiotic eardrops, but may require surgical removal. This lengthy procedure, performed under general anaesthetic, often requires an incision behind the ear or through the ear canal opening. Cyst infections must be treated to prevent recurrence, hearing loss, balance disturbance and other complications.

Continued on p166 ▶

communication skills

When we speak to someone, the words we use play a surprisingly small part in what we understand from the conversation. Tone of voice and body language are probably just as important to our grasp of what's being said.

An audiologist will be keen to make sure that you are using all your communication skills to your best advantage and that both you and your family know how best to compensate for any hearing loss. Some local hospitals even run communications skills courses. Meanwhile here are some tips:

- The best distance at which to hold a conversation is 1-2m (3-6ft). Don't try to talk to someone from a distance or, worse, from the next room.

For people with hearing loss, lip-reading and hearing aids work together to improve communication abilities.

- If you need glasses, wear them.
- Make sure you can see the other person's face full on, especially their lips.
- If you have better hearing in one ear than the other, position yourself so the other person is on your 'good' side.
- Watch the other person's face, gestures, posture and body movements – you can get a lot of clues about what they're saying from aspects other than speech.

- If you're not sure you've heard correctly, don't ask someone to repeat the words, ask them to say it in a different way. Or try a technique called reverse questioning to confirm (or otherwise). 'So I'll see you at 2 o'clock then?' or 'goodness, it took how long?'
- Try to stay calm. No one hears correctly all the time, and if you become anxious or flustered you may miss more. If it's noisy, ask if you can talk in a quieter place.

LIP-READING

Most of us lip-read to some extent when we're having a conversation against background noise – such as in a noisy bar – though we might not realise we're doing it. It helps to 'fill in the gaps' in speech, especially if we have some idea what's being discussed. For people with hearing loss, lip-reading and hearing aids work together to improve communication abilities.

Your audiologist will probably know about local courses – they may even be run in the hospital. If you have a mild hearing impairment, lip-reading can help a great deal to compensate for sounds that you may otherwise miss during a conversation. For people with a severe hearing impairment, lip-reading may be the best or only way to communicate in everyday situations.

But it is more difficult to be a skilled lip-reader than you might think. Many letters and words produce the same mouth shapes when spoken. For example, 'park', 'bark' and 'mark' all look the same, and even words that sound completely different – sometimes with opposite meanings, like 'red' and 'green' – are mouthed in a similar way.

A year of weekly classes is usually enough for most people to get a good grasp of the principles, and many people find that it makes a huge difference. Indeed, 'for the majority of active adults', says the Association of Teachers of Lipreading to Adults, 'it may be the most important element in their rehabilitation'. See the Resources section, pages 238-241, for information on finding a local class.

PLEASE DO THIS – ADVICE TO FRIENDS AND RELATIVES

If you can't hear what's being said, you can feel isolated. Your family and friends could help to minimise this – so if your hearing isn't as good as it was, copy out this list and stick it somewhere obvious. And if you're reading this because someone you care about has a hearing problem, take careful note as these measures will help.

- Make sure you have my attention before you start speaking.
- Try to stand or sit about 1m (3ft) away and facing the light, so that I can see your face clearly.
- Turn your face directly towards me when you talk to me, so that I can see your mouth movements. Even with a hearing aid, I can't pick up everything you say.
- Speak as clearly as you can, but don't talk too slowly or simplify what you say – I have a problem with hearing, not with my capacity to understand.
- Don't shout! Raising your voice can distort the sound and make it more difficult to identify individual words. It may also be painful, especially if I am wearing a hearing aid. In public, it's embarrassing.
- If I don't follow what you have said, try saying it again in a different way.
- Keep your hands away from your mouth, and don't chew while you are talking. If we are together a lot, please shave off your beard or moustache. Obscuring your mouth makes it much harder to lip-read.
- Turn off the TV and other background noise when we talk.

gadgets and gizmos

Modern technology has made life much easier for people with hearing impairment. You can opt to watch most TV programmes with subtitles. Everyday gadgets convey information visually as well as through sound – look at text messages on mobile phones and email. And most mobile phones can be set to vibrate instead of ring.

Assistive Listening Devices (ALDs) based on induction loops, infrared or radio signals are increasingly available in banks, shops, museums, theatres and other venues, and can also be used in workplaces, schools and colleges. They augment standard public address and audio systems by providing signals that can be received either by means of special receivers that eliminate or filter background noise or through your own hearing aid.

There's also a wide range of gadgets available to use in the home to make up for reduced hearing, either by boosting sound levels or by providing some sort of alternative alerting system. Here are a few examples:

- Doorbells with sound amplifiers or flashing lights.
- Door beacons that react to the vibration of knocking to set off a flashing light.
- Phone amplifiers with adjustable extra volume.
- Flashing and vibrating alarm clocks.
- Vibrating wrist-watches.
- Vibrating pagers, alert systems and timers.
- Ear-hooks that eliminate interference from mobile phones.
- Baby monitors with visual alerts.
- A portable pager that flashes in response to signals from your doorbell, phone, smoke alarm or baby monitor.
- Personal listening devices that allow you to listen to the TV at a volume that suits you, without affecting other users.

cutting EDGE

TEXT RADIO

It may seem counter-intuitive for someone who can't hear to be able to enjoy speech-based radio programmes, but it could well be possible in the near future. A system that converts voice to text in real time is being developed by a US consortium of communications company Harris Corporation, National Public Radio and Towson University in Maryland. The technique involves broadcasting a text translation simultaneously with a digital radio programme, for display on a screen incorporated into the radio – similar to 'closed captioning' systems for television. The translation is done by keyboard operators at present, but could one day be performed automatically.

- Television captioning (available on newer sets).
- Fire alarms that set off a powerful flashing light or a vibrating pad you keep under your pillow.
- Loop systems for home TV, radio and hi-fi.

Most of these are available through specialist suppliers. The RNID, for example, has its own online shop – www.rnid.org.uk/shop – and also reviews new products.

turn off
that mute button

Even if you only have a small amount of hearing loss it's worth considering one of the new generation of hearing aids. There are hundreds of different types and models, and your audiologist will help you to choose which is best for you. All hearing aids have a microphone, an amplifier, a receiver (like a miniature loudspeaker), a battery and a made-to-measure ear mould.

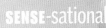
FURRY FRIENDS

One alternative to gadgets is a hearing dog. Just like guide dogs for the blind, these dogs are trained to alert their owners to specific sounds, like alarm clocks, doorbells, phones or smoke alarms. Hearing dogs can provide welcome company and a degree of vital independence for anyone with severe hearing loss. You can find details in our Resources section.

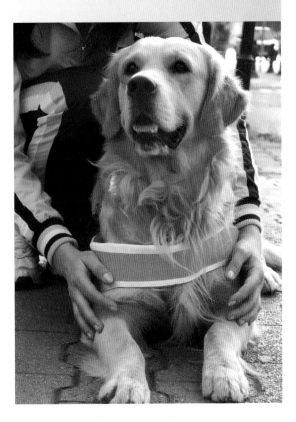

IT'S A DIGITAL WORLD

All NHS audiology departments offer digital hearing aids. These are vastly superior to the old analogue sort – better at eliminating background noise and whistle, and programmable to manage sounds of different volumes to suit you. While the NHS aims to treat within 18 weeks, there may still be waiting lists for aids, though you can buy them privately – at a price.

When you get your new hearing aid your audiologist will adjust the settings so that different sounds are always heard at levels that are comfortable for you. But it can take several visits before your aid fits and works just right. Some aids allow you to switch between different settings for different conditions; others automatically self-adjust to different sound environments. Some aids improve your ability to hear clearly in noisy situations by incorporating directional microphones, which amplify sounds selectively from one direction. And some have a T setting that picks up signals from a loop system or hearing aid-compatible telephone.

WHERE DO YOU WEAR IT?

Aids can be broadly categorised according to where you wear them – behind the ear or in the ear. Some specialist aids conduct sound through bone instead of air.

BEHIND-THE-EAR (BTE) AIDS

These are the most common type of NHS aids. An ear mould inside your ear transmits sounds, while the rest of the device sits behind your ear, with a plastic tube connecting it to the ear mould. It can be programmed and coupled to other devices such as phones and loop systems.

A new version, called an open ear fitting, has a smaller, softer earpiece that doesn't require an ear mould – so it's less conspicuous – and it can give a very natural sound. These are usually suitable only for milder forms of hearing loss, but some types can be used for quite severe loss and can then be modified to include a mould if hearing becomes worse and you need more help.

BONE-CONDUCTING HEARING AIDS

These are used when someone cannot wear conventional aids or has such severe conductive hearing loss that sound cannot be transmitted through the ear canal. A small bone vibrator sits behind the ear and sends sound vibrations through the skull, which are detected directly in the inner ear.

Bone-conducting hearing aids can be held in place with a headband, or you can have a safe operation to implant a 'bone anchored' aid permanently. It avoids the discomfort of wearing a headband and the sound result is vastly superior, as sound is transmitted directly to the bone without having to go through skin and tissue. Bone-conducting hearing aids are available on the NHS in specialist units.

IN-THE-EAR (ITE) AIDS

Sometimes called 'custom' hearing aids, these are small enough for all the gadgetry to fit inside the ear mould, which then sits inside your ear – so they are less noticeable than BTE aids. Some fill up the outer ear so can be seen from the outside, but the smallest fit right inside the ear canal and are

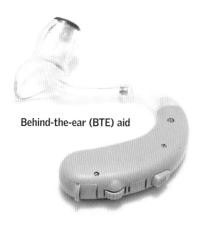

Behind-the-ear (BTE) aid

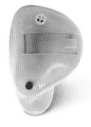

In-the-ear (ITE) aid

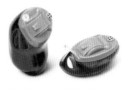

In-the-ear (ITE) aid

Hearing aids The BTE aid is one of the most common hearing aids but custom aids, such as the ITE types above, are less conspicuous – especially the smallest ones (above right), which fit into the ear canal.

Even if you only have a small amount of hearing loss it's worth considering one of the new generation of hearing aids.

almost invisible – a huge advantage if you are embarrassed or self conscious about needing a hearing aid, though they are much more fiddly to insert and operate.

ITE aids are not suitable for everyone. You may not be able to use one if you have very narrow ear canals, and in general the greater your degree of hearing loss, the larger your aid needs to be. Because some ITE devices are very small, it may not be possible to have a T setting.

COCHLEAR IMPLANTS – 'BIONIC EARS'

Unlike hearing aids, cochlear implants work not by amplifying sound but by directly stimulating the auditory nerve inside the inner ear through a surgically-implanted electronic device. They are often called 'bionic ears' but the hearing they provide is not exactly normal but more the 'sensation' of sound, though many who use them interpret the sound well enough to converse on the phone. Provided the auditory nerve is still functioning, they can make a huge difference to people with profound hearing impairment for whom hearing aid amplification is insufficient, and are increasingly being offered to adults as well as children.

Implants can be life-changing. In adults, depending on the duration of deafness, they can help people return to work and a near normal home life. Given early enough to children born deaf, they can enable them to develop good speech and language, enjoy normal schooling and even university education.

If you get little or no benefit from a hearing aid, you may qualify for an implant on the NHS. The operation is carried out under general anaesthetic and usually involves two or three days in hospital. The implant itself

Continued on p173 ➤

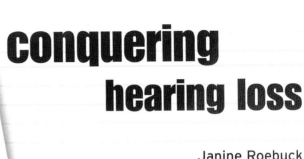

conquering hearing loss

Janine Roebuck

It's hard to imagine that anyone who is deaf could triumph on stage as an opera singer, and indeed for many years Janine Roebuck kept her problem a virtual secret, afraid that admitting it would be a handicap when she auditioned for roles.

Janine was 18 when she learned that she had inherited an incurable form of progressive nerve deafness, which had affected several generations of her family. 'My great-great-grandmother had been born stone deaf. Six or seven of her 13 children inherited the gene; the others didn't,' Janine says. 'My father and I, both only children, drew the short straw.'

As a child, unaware of the hearing difficulties that lay in wait for her, she had joined Doncaster Youth Theatre and discovered the joys of acting and singing. Aged 13, she sang a principal role in a school opera. 'From the moment the curtains opened on the first night, I knew without the shadow of a doubt how I wanted to spend the rest of my life.'

At her parents' urging, she first went to university and obtained a degree in French Studies before focusing on singing. 'I first noticed I had a hearing problem in university lectures, particularly if I wasn't lucky enough to bag a front row seat. I was forever looking over my friend's shoulder to see what she'd written. Initial consonants were the first to go, and that is still a major problem on the phone today, despite amplification, as I rely heavily on lip-reading.'

DEVASTATING NEWS

At university she performed with the university's opera group, which happened to be run by an audiology professor. Janine asked him if he would test her father.

'As the case was such an interesting one, they tested me too and bang – the news I'd dreaded.'

'Enjoy singing as much as you can now,' she was told, 'because with your hearing loss, there's absolutely no way you could have a career in music.'

'I was utterly devastated,' Janine says. 'I went for a private consultation with one of the singing teachers at the Royal Northern College of Music, who was the second person to tell me I should just keep on singing as a hobby. I was heartbroken and sobbed all the way home on the bus.'

But her determination to become an opera singer was so all-consuming that she refused to listen to the doom-merchants. 'I thought there was a chance that, by the time I needed it, technology might have improved sufficiently to help me.'

AGAINST THE ODDS

She got top marks in her first singing examination, went on to study at the Paris Conservatoire and the National Opera Studio, then made her debut with New Sadler's Wells Opera. She has since sung principal roles with many first-class opera companies and appeared at major venues both in Britain and abroad – including the Royal Opera House – and has many CD recordings to her credit.

Janine was about 28 when the inevitable deterioration in her hearing became a problem. 'I noticed it most at first in little things, for instance, in rehearsals one day the room suddenly went very quiet and I realised with a sickening thud that the director had been talking to me and I hadn't heard him.' On another occasion, when she was singing a title role on tour in a venue where the orchestra was under the stage, and there were no speakers on stage or in the wings, a reviewer queried whether she could hear the orchestra at all. 'He had no idea just how true that was.'

But her first hearing aid did little to improve things. 'It amplified even the frequencies that didn't need enhancing, which was uncomfortable,' says Janine. 'I left the hearing aid in a drawer and was too terrified to mention my deafness to a soul, afraid they would see me as too much of a liability to employ me.'

MIRACULOUS TECHNOLOGY

Then, by chance, she saw a professor at London's Royal National Ear, Nose and Throat Hospital, who referred her to 'a superb audiological scientist'. He gave her two behind-the-ear analogue hearing aids, computer generated to ensure that only the upper frequencies that she had lost were amplified – and coloured brown, to blend with her hair.

'I heard birds sing and the sound of high heels clicking on pavements for the first time in ten years. It made me weep for joy, although the sound was very artificial at first.' The technician promised her that her brain would get used to the harsh mechanical sound and would adjust to make it seem more normal – which is exactly what happened.

'I heard birds sing and the sound of high heels clicking on pavements for the first time in ten years. It made me weep for joy.'

But Janine still had problems. 'My behind-the-ear hearing aids used to catch on my stage wigs and whistle, or unhook at the unlikeliest moments and dangle over my ear like a tiny rear view mirror, making me blush with shame.'

Eventually she decided to pay privately for a pair of tiny, analogue in-ear hearing aids. Without them, she believes 'I certainly wouldn't be singing today. They were worth every penny.' She continues to seek out the latest technology and now has two digital aids called Epoq, made by Oticon, which use bluetooth technology. 'I am absolutely thrilled with them,' she says. 'They have given me a quality of sound I hitherto only dreamed of.'

RISING TO THE CHALLENGE

There are still huge obstacles, especially in a musical career. Janine can't always hear what an audition panel is saying, which can lead to amusing misunderstandings, and has

'I can sleep soundly in noisy hotel rooms on tour – even through rowdy guests or discos.'

difficulty if the conductor and orchestra are behind her on stage in a concert, as visual cues are vital to her. All this can create great anxiety. But there are plus points, too. 'I have to sing by sensation, not by listening to myself, so I sing from the heart. People have commented that I sing with real feeling, that my voice moves them, even makes them cry with emotion. It gives me the greatest joy to be told that.'

Another advantage is being able to turn down the volume. 'I can turn the hearing aids off if I want some hush. That means I can sleep soundly in noisy hotel rooms on tour – even through rowdy guests or discos – though I was once nearly burnt to a crisp in a hotel through not hearing the fire alarm. Now I notify people that I would need rescuing if an emergency arose during the night.'

A CRUSADE IN THE MAKING

Janine's experience has made her determined to highlight the awful isolation that deafness can bring. 'I have a burning desire to help ensure that the elderly, particularly those in hospital, have their hearing aids checked daily,' she says. 'Often people get too confused to realise they are not working properly or need new batteries, and just think that their hearing has deteriorated. What often happens is that nurses turn them off or put them in a drawer if they whistle and disturb the other patients. Or the ear moulds become loose because someone has lost weight, and no-one thinks to replace them. This can result in a frightened, lonely, deaf patient being treated as senile and stupid, simply because he or she is cut off and isolated.

'I'm no longer ashamed of my deafness. I feel it has helped to make me strong. It has taught me that if you are determined enough, anything can be surmounted, and that's a message I want to pass on to other people.'

consists of electrodes inserted into the cochlea, which will be 'switched on' at a later stage. In addition, a tiny receiver incorporating a magnet is inserted under the skin above and behind your ear – the magnet is to make sure that the external transmitter remains in place directly beside the implanted receiver. To use the implant, you need to wear a transmitter coil behind your ear along with a microphone and speech processor either behind the ear, like a hearing aid, or in a small box that can be clipped elsewhere, such as to a waistband. The microphone picks up environmental sounds and converts them to electrical signals, which are sent via the processor to the transmitter. The electrodes in the implant detect these and stimulate the hair cells in the cochlea to send signals down the auditory nerve, as in natural hearing.

When the device is switched on it can take a while for your brain to learn to interpret the signals as distinct sounds, but you will soon become aware of environmental noises, such as alarms and doorbells, and learn to distinguish between them. Although the quality of sound is not normal, implants bring your hearing sensitivity to normal levels.

A great benefit is that you'll be able to tell immediately when someone is talking, which can help you to follow speech in conjunction with lip-reading. It also enables you to 'hear' how loudly you are speaking, which can be a great help in conversation. Some people get good enough sound quality to allow them to understand speech directly and have near normal conversations as long as there's no background noise. Above all the cochlear implant has given people hope, says ENT specialist Matthew Yung. 'What many patients find reassuring is that with implants now there is virtually no level of hearing loss that cannot be improved.'

your smart sense plan

Within the preceding pages are all the elements you need to put your *Smart Sense Plan* for hearing into action. You know how to Protect your hearing from the dangers of noise that surround us, and all about the healthy diet and lifestyle that's as good for your ears as it is for your eyes. You've learned to Assess your hearing level and understand how to spot the symptoms of reduced hearing and other ear problems – and you know where to go for help if you need it. You have discovered how medical treatment can help hearing problems and other symptoms, and how the wonders of modern technology are making life so much better for people with hearing impairments. You know just how much can be done to Correct any problems that arise. So now it's time to Enjoy the pleasures of sharp hearing for life.

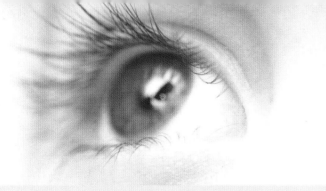
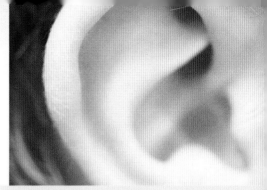

11 your smart hearing plan

If you've read through this section, you'll now know a great deal about hearing and what you can do to protect and preserve it. You'll understand how the incredibly delicate structures in your ear work – and how easy it is to damage them. You'll also be aware, that it's a mistake to ignore changes that could suggest a hearing problem, because there is so much that can be done to treat, reverse or compensate for any hearing loss. **So here are a few reminders to help you to ensure that your Smart Sense Plan for hearing will safeguard this precious sense, and allow you to enjoy the sounds of life, for life.**

Protect your ears

- Are you regularly exposed to loud noise? 118-119, 127-128
- Do you do anything to limit your noise exposure? 131
- Have you bought earplugs to use in especially noisy situations? 129
- If your workplace is noisy, do you wear the ear defenders provided? 129
- Do you smoke? If so, have you sought help to stop? 130
- Are your blood pressure and cholesterol under control? 133
- And are you following your doctor's recommendations if you have heart disease or diabetes? 130
- Do you regularly eat salty foods and add table salt? 133
- Do you also know how eating cheese, butter and fatty meat can affect your hearing? 133
- Do you eat plenty of fruit and vegetables? 132-136
- Do you get enough sunshine or vitamin D-containing foods? 135

Assess your ears

- Do you know the signs of a possible hearing problem? 117
- Did you know that you could take a telephone or internet hearing test? (But do also see your GP and get a formal assessment, if necessary.) 123
- Is your balance sense as good as it was? 124
- Do you have difficult hearing some speech sounds such as - 's', 'th', 'ch' and 'f, or 'p', 'k' and 't'? 141

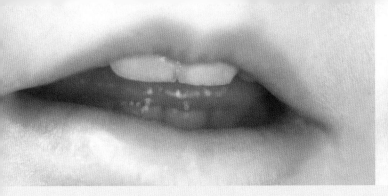
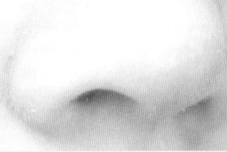

- Do you understand the symptoms of common ear conditions? 144
- Do you have ringing in the ears or other unwanted noises? 149
- Do you have episodes of giddiness? 150

Correct any problems

- Do you know which symptoms suggest you should seek immediate help? 144
- Have you arranged to see your GP about any hearing problems or related symptoms? 153
- Do you know why it is important to have early treatment? 140
- Have you asked your GP if any medicines or drugs you're taking could be causing your ear symptoms? 146-147
- Do you understand how hearing tests diagnose a problem? 154-155
- Are you aware of the sophisticated range of hearing aids available? 167-169
- Do you know the best techniques for communicating if you have hearing impairment? 164-165
- Are you aware of all the gadgets and gizmos now available to help people with impaired hearing? 166-167

Enjoy your sense of hearing

- Which sounds give you the greatest pleasure? Often it's the voices of the people you love – husband, children, parents. Perhaps you could make recordings to keep of the people you cherish.
- When you listen to music, see if you can pick out different instruments or voices. Listen carefully; this is a skill you can improve.
- If you enjoy birdsong, buy a birdsong CD and learn to identify the birds that visit your garden or neighbourhood.
- What other noises make you happy? Often it's evocative sounds, such as church bells on a summer's evening, children's laughter as they play outside, rain pattering on the roof of a canvas tent or marquee, the rustle of leaves as you walk in autumn woods.
- From time to time, take a moment or two simply to stand still and listen – whether in the garden, out in the park, on a beach or enjoying a walk in the country. What can you hear?

Taste &

These senses have an important role to play, tempting us to eat and drink the vital nutrients our bodies need, or warning us of poisons and other dangers. They also add such pleasure to our lives that there is every incentive to protect and even enhance them.

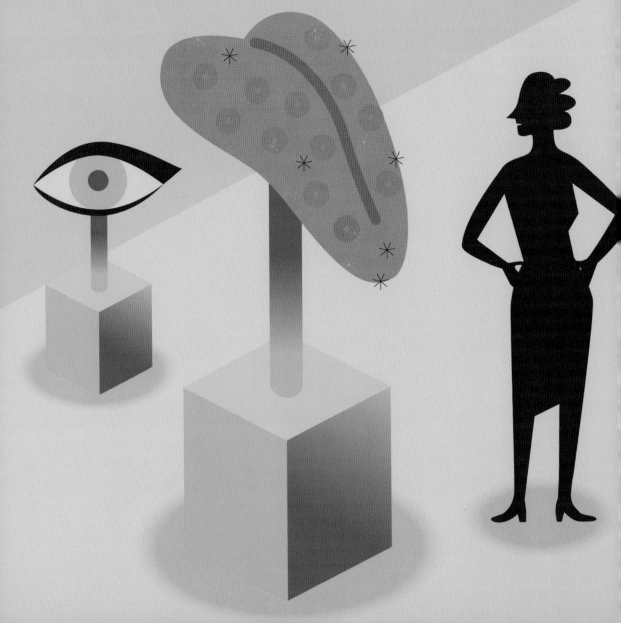

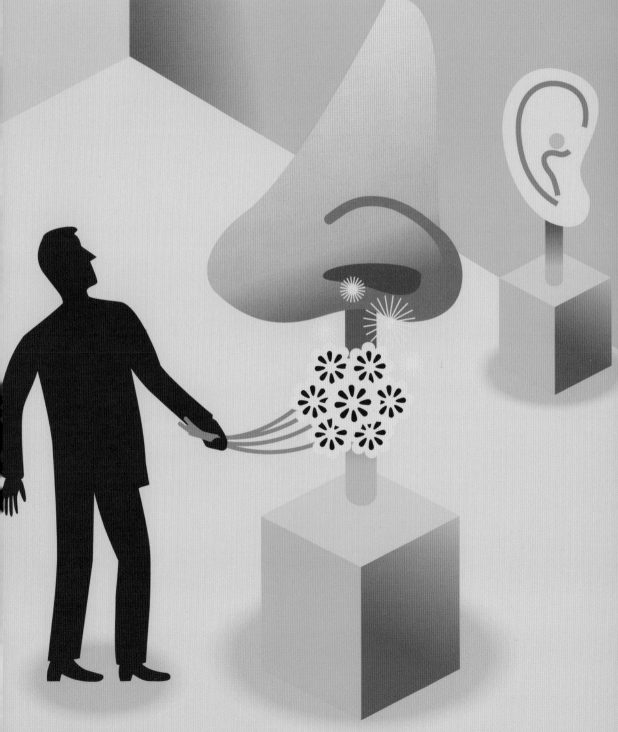

smell

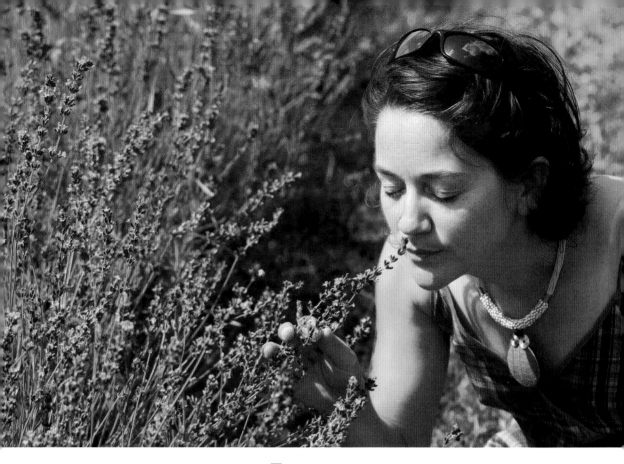

12

The spice of life

Think about the delicious sensation of chocolate as it melts in your mouth, the salty tang of seaside air, the aroma of fresh coffee or the fragrance of lavender, lilac or honeysuckle wafting across a garden.

Our ability to taste or to smell may not appear to be as important to our well-being as sight or hearing, or to affect our safety, independence, work or relationships in quite the same way. But, as you'll learn in this section, these, too, are senses that we should not take for granted as both influence important aspects of our lives in vital and enjoyable ways.

Taste and smell enhance our enjoyment of everyday things. Your *Smart Sense Plan* is not simply about being safe, independent and able to function – an earthworm in the right location can have all those. It is also about relishing all the good things that life has to offer. And, although our sense of smell is vastly inferior to that of many animals, we still use it as a form of communication, frequently unconsciously. Smell can, in fact, help you to detect the emotions of those around you and it undoubtedly influences your choice of sexual partner. It may trigger memories, or affect your mood and even your immune system and hormonal balance.

vital role

All our lives, taste and smell will influence what we eat and drink. And, interestingly, most people find that some foods taste and even smell different at different ages. As we grow up and our tastes mature, we become better able to savour foods that we may have hated as a child, such as dark chocolate or strong cheeses. We often become less fussy, but more discerning – delighting in sampling foods from different regions and cultures, for instance, or developing a taste for fine wines.

But these glorious senses did not, in fact, develop primarily to enable us to delight in lobster thermidor, a glass of Merlot or a bacon sandwich, or to savour the aroma of freshly-baked bread or new-mown grass – however kind it is of nature to have organised it so that we can. Like our other senses, they evolved to protect us from unseen dangers, such as poison or a smouldering fire, and to help us to survive. It's not for nothing that things that are foul-smelling or taste revolting are often hazardous to eat.

WHY THEY MATTER

There is no doubt that our sense of taste and smell tends to decline as we get older. Since the decline is not obviously life-threatening, people pay it much less attention than the deterioration of other senses. But it is potentially dangerous. People with reduced taste sensation have to be more careful about what they eat because they are more vulnerable to food poisoning. Those whose sense of smell is impaired are more at risk from a gas leak or a fire hazard that others could usually detect.

And declining taste and smell can have other health implications. For example, older people with fading smell and taste sensations, who no longer enjoy food as much as they did when they were younger, may lose interest in meals and eat less than they should. This can result in

WHY DO BAD THINGS TASTE SO GOOD?

We all know that crispy salads and brown rice are good for us, but most people have at some time regretted that such 'healthy' foods don't have quite the same taste impact as, say, bacon and eggs, or chips or cream cakes. But why not? Well, in the days when humans had to forage or hunt for everything they ate, eating high-energy foods – those high in fats or sugars – was the healthy option, as it gave people a survival advantage when food was scarce. So we are programmed by evolution to want foods that pile on the calories, and our taste buds haven't caught up with the fact that the problem is that now there is often too much food available.

nutritional deficiencies – which in turn can exacerbate smell and taste disorders, creating a vicious circle. People who are able to distinguish the tastes of only those foods that are fatty and calorific – and not subtle tastes – could easily become overweight; loss of sensation does not cause the weight gain, but it can be an associated factor. Similarly, people who are losing their sense of taste may make a habit of adding salt to their meals to heighten the flavour – and excessive quantities of salt can increase the risk of high blood pressure. This could set up another type of vicious circle, since high blood pressure is one of several conditions that can actually promote smell or taste disorders.

ENEMIES OF SMELL AND TASTE

Almost all of us find that there are certain times in our lives when we cannot smell or taste as well as normal. Below is a list of everyday factors that can cause this deficiency.

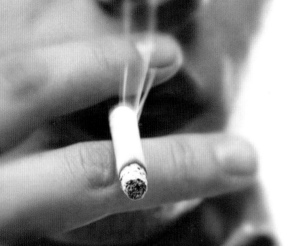

- Colds and other respiratory infections
- Hay fever (rhinitis) and other allergies
- Sinus conditions
- Nasal polyps
- Dental disease
- Diabetes
- High blood pressure
- Side effects of some medications
- Smoking
- Poor diet
- Vitamin deficiency

Smoking is one of the enemies of smell and taste.

There are other illnesses and accidents that can have a major impact on taste and smell – head injuries, brain tumours, Alzheimer's disease, schizophrenia and neurological disorders such as multiple sclerosis or Parkinson's disease, as well as exposure to chemicals, toxins or radiation. Exposure to certain harmful substances may be unavoidable. But you will realise that at least some of the risk factors listed are within your control. As part of your *Smart Sense Plan* you will learn what you can do to minimise or treat the underlying condition. You can probably already think of some ways to Protect your taste and smell senses – the first step of your **PACE** strategy; the next chapter will explain several more.

BE ALERT TO CHANGES

As you go through this section, you'll learn more about how you can help to preserve these precious senses, about the causes of smell and taste disorders, and what can be done to treat them. The message here is never to ignore reduced, distorted, or lost sensations of taste or smell, nor accept them as an inevitable feature of getting older – not least because they may alert your doctor to other potentially treatable problems.

People with impaired smell and taste also have an impaired quality of life. As well as losing interest in food, you may cut back on going out to eat or inviting friends over for a meal, or even popping next door for a coffee. A lunch at your local pub or a snack in your favourite café no longer seem so tempting. A hobby such as gardening might lose some of its appeal if you can't smell the fragrant flowers that you're growing. And your home may be less welcoming to others if you can't detect and banish unpleasant odours, such as the smell of pets or stale cooking.

So although they may not seem as crucial to your well-being as sight and hearing, paying attention to smell and taste is an important part of your *Smart Sense Plan*. This chapter explains how these senses work together to provide so much enjoyment in life.

smell and taste – the intimate link

It may seem obvious that smelling is carried out by the nose and tasting by the mouth. But actually much of your sensation of *flavour*, and thus your enjoyment of food, comes through your sense of smell. That's why you often can't taste food properly when you have a cold and a blocked nose. The flavour of some foods, such as chocolate or coffee, is almost entirely dependent on smell – a phenomenon explained below.

Although people often use the words taste and flavour interchangeably to mean the same thing, the flavour of food is actually made up of taste and smell. Sense experts estimate that at least 75 per cent of what we perceive as taste actually arises from our sense of smell.

When you eat grated apple, the taste buds alone would have difficulty distinguishing it from grated onion.

That is why medical specialists report that people almost never complain that they have lost their sense of smell, but tend to say that they can't taste their food properly any more.

What's more, while the taste buds on your tongue can distinguish five distinct taste sensations (see page 186), the smell receptors in your nose can distinguish hundreds of odours, even if they are only subtly different or present only in tiny amounts, sometimes at concentrations as low as a few parts per trillion. Your sense of smell is 10,000 times more sensitive than your sense of taste.

TWO TYPES OF SMELLING

The process of smelling, known medically as 'olfaction', occurs in two ways. As well as the type of smelling that occurs when you sniff something, called orthonasal olfaction, scientists have found that a second form of smelling kicks in when you eat, as odours from swallowed food are pushed back up through passages between the mouth and the nose to reach the smell receptors at the top of the nose. This is known as retronasal olfaction, and it is partly responsible for the link between smell and taste sensations.

When you eat grated apple, your taste buds alone would have difficulty distinguishing it from grated onion. (In a test like this, both foods are grated so that they have a similar texture and mouth-feel.) But, as the apple or onion mixes with saliva in your mouth, odour molecules are released that travel from the back of the throat up into the nasal passages, where, based on past memories, the food is correctly identified. Retronasal olfaction enables you to appreciate full flavour. Or, try holding your nose before chewing on a sweet. After a couple of seconds, release your nose – what you experience is the difference between taste and flavour.

SENSE-sational

IT GETS THE DIGESTIVE JUICES FLOWING

Even before you sit down to eat, your nose – by means of orthonasal olfaction – helps to initiate digestion. You sniff the aroma of eagerly anticipated food, which triggers saliva secretion in preparation for the process by which your body will break down starch in the food.

smelling step-by-step

Olfaction is carried out by specialised receptor cells. These are essentially nerve cells with long hairs called cilia projecting from one end.

1 Odour molecules carried on the air pass over the olfactory region within the nasal cavity.

2 The odour molecules dissolve in the mucus that lines the nasal cavity.

3 The molecules reach receptor cells specialised to respond to their particular odour and bind to the receptor molecules on the surface of the receptor cell, triggering a response.

4 The receptor cell sends a nerve signal to the brain.

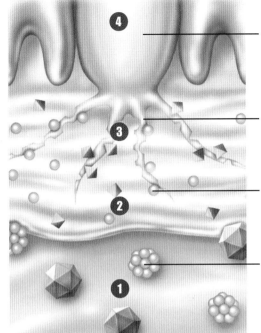

Apical knob Each receptor cell is capped with a raised apical knob that projects very slightly through the surface of the olfactory region.

Cilia Sprouting out of each apical knob are around 10 to 20 whip-like filaments called cilia, each 0.0001mm wide. Cilia increase the surface area to which odour molecules can bind.

Odour molecule dissolved in the mucus that lines the nasal cavity.

Odour molecules carried along within inhaled air.

The two types of smelling – orthonasal and retronasal – are curiously distinct. Sniffing through the nose gives you no sensation of flavour at all, whereas retronasal olfaction becomes stronger with a greater intensity of sensation from within the mouth when you start eating. The two processes are experienced quite differently – think, for example, of the difference between smelling ripe cheese from across the room and the impression of flavour you get from actually eating it.

CHEMICAL SENSES

The senses of smell and taste differ from vision and hearing because they require direct physical contact in order to impart information about the outside world. We smell because our noses detect odour molecules carried in the air, and we taste only when food molecules dissolve in saliva to be detected by sensory receptors in our mouths.

Unlike vision and hearing, smell and taste are chemical senses – they rely on specialised receptor cells that are stimulated by molecules dissolving in the fluid surrounding them – saliva in the mouth and mucus in the nose. While taste receptors can only sense substances actually in the mouth, smells may waft into the nose on the air from some distance away, depending on wind direction and other factors.

an intricate
smelling machine

At the top of the nose is a small area about the size of a postage stamp called the olfactory epithelium – the smelling surface. Into this tiny area are packed millions of receptor cells called olfactory receptor neurones. Each cell has a number of hair-like projections called cilia hanging downwards into the nasal cavity, covered in thin, clear mucus. Odours reach the nose in the form of airborne molecules that then dissolve in this mucus, enabling receptors in the cilia to respond.

Our smell sensitivity is generally lowest first thing in the morning, and improves as the day goes on; it's also stronger in spring and summer than at other times of the year.

If the mucus becomes so thick that it can no longer dissolve the molecules from the air – which happens when you have a cold – you lose your sense of smell.

Impulses from the receptors travel along olfactory nerve fibres to the olfactory bulbs, one for each nostril, which sit behind the nose just underneath the brain. Incoming information is processed in the bulbs and sent to the smell centre, called the olfactory area, in the brain, where smell sensations are interpreted.

The olfactory region is unusual in that it connects directly to the limbic system – a group of deep brain structures, that play an important part in the regulation of human moods and

SENSE-sational

SNIFFING OUT SUPPER

Your ability to smell is boosted when you're hungry – presumably a throwback to the days when humans had to forage and hunt their own food, and being able to sniff out supper would have provided a survival advantage.

emotions; this may help to explain why we find that certain smells instantly trigger a range of memories and associations (see page 190).

Odour recognition is a complex process – the brain must analyse more than 300 different molecules in order to identify the fragrance of a rose, for example. Smell sensitivity is generally lowest first thing in the morning, and improves as the day goes on; it's also stronger in spring and summer than at other times of the year.

the sense of smell

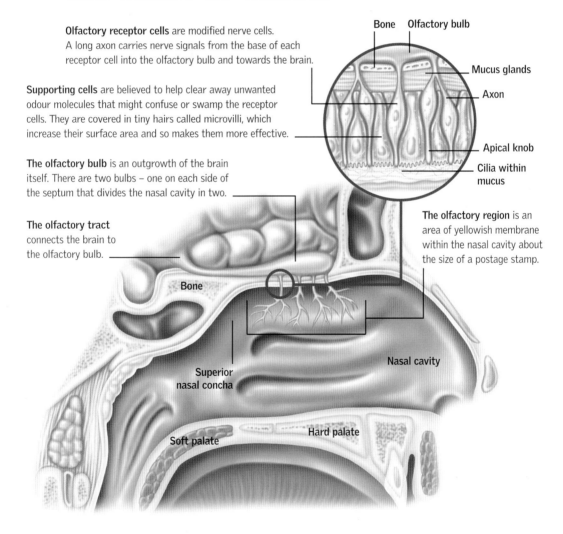

Olfactory receptor cells are modified nerve cells. A long axon carries nerve signals from the base of each receptor cell into the olfactory bulb and towards the brain.

Supporting cells are believed to help clear away unwanted odour molecules that might confuse or swamp the receptor cells. They are covered in tiny hairs called microvilli, which increase their surface area and so makes them more effective.

The olfactory bulb is an outgrowth of the brain itself. There are two bulbs – one on each side of the septum that divides the nasal cavity in two.

The olfactory tract connects the brain to the olfactory bulb.

Bone   Olfactory bulb

Mucus glands

Axon

Apical knob

Cilia within mucus

The olfactory region is an area of yellowish membrane within the nasal cavity about the size of a postage stamp.

Bone

Superior nasal concha

Nasal cavity

Soft palate

Hard palate

how you taste

You probably learned a little about taste buds in biology classes at school – that they are the tiny sensory organs which detect different taste sensations amd are housed in all those bumps, or papillae, on the tongue.

You may also have learnt that they enable you to identify four basic tastes – sweet, sour, salty and bitter – and that all taste sensations result from a combination of these fundamental tastes. Some years ago, it was common scientific wisdom that the taste buds for each of these were located in different areas of the tongue – sweet on the tip, salty on either

The flavour common to asparagus, tomatoes, cheese and meat is distinctively different from the traditional four tastes.

side towards the front, sour on either side towards the back, and bitter right at the back.

SEAWEED SENSATION

Much of this thinking has changed. Scientists now recognise that there are five basic taste sensations. The fifth, known as umami (pronounced yu-mah-mee), was named nearly a century ago by a Japanese scientist, Professor Kikunae Ikeda, who realised that a particular flavour common to asparagus, tomatoes, cheese and meat was distinctively different from the traditional four tastes. There is no precise English translation for umami; the nearest equivalent is 'deliciousness', but it may be described as savoury or meaty.

The taste has been recognised for centuries in Oriental cuisine. It occurs in a broth made from kombu, a type of seaweed, from which Prof. Ikeda succeeded in extracting the substance that creates the taste - glutamate. This is an amino acid, a building block of protein molecules. Glutamate is present naturally in almost all foods, and in high concentrations in a wide variety of foods commonly regarded as especially tasty, including meat, fish, duck, dairy products, mushrooms, ripe tomatoes (especially beefsteak tomatoes), sugar snap peas, grapefruit, tea, ginger and tofu. There are especially high levels in Parmesan cheese, bacon and cured prosciutto.

But despite Prof. Ikeda's discovery, the fifth taste was largely ignored by Western scientists until recent years. But the seasoning that he developed from glutamate, monosodium glutamate (MSG), made his fortune and is widely used throughout the world – especially in Chinese restaurants in the UK. Then, in 1996, researchers at the University of Miami discovered separate taste receptors for umami in the tongue. Since the research was published in 2000, umami has become much more widely known and is now accepted as one of the five basic taste sensations.

WRONG THINKING

Scientists also recognise that the taste-bud map is also an over-simplification, based on a misunderstanding. It was originally thought that where a certain taste sensation on the tongue was felt most strongly, other tastes could not be detected and, for some reason, the fallacy persisted for more than 100 years. Yet it's easy to show that the 'map' doesn't work – just put a bit of salt on the tip of your tongue: it still tastes salty.

In fact, the five basic tastes – and there may be more – can be detected all over the tongue, except for a small 'bald' patch at the centre of the tongue, which has few papillae. There are also some variations in sensitivity – for example, there may be more bitter taste receptors than others to warn against noxious foods – but these differences are relatively insignificant.

SO GOOD TO EAT!

The presence of glutamate greatly enhances the taste of food, and scientists speculate that our bodies developed the ability to recognise its taste specifically because umami signals a high-protein food, essential for survival. This would explain why we tend to crave foods with high levels of natural glutamate.

Some top chefs are using this new knowledge to create umami-packed dishes in restaurants. It is also helping efforts by the food industry to cut back on fat, salt, sugar and artificial ingredients in response to consumer demand: high-umami foods offer high flavour without the drawbacks of unhealthy additives.

But umami has also been branded a villain because it makes high fat foods such as pizza and crisps taste so good. And, it has been claimed that the use of MSG (glutamate extracted from food sources and used as a seasoning) in some fast food meals makes them 'addictive' and so contributes to weight gain.

Clearly, ultra-delicious tastes have drawbacks in countries where processed food is over-plentiful and obesity rates are soaring.

how taste buds work

You can't actually see taste buds – they're much too small. They sit on the top or sides of the little bumps, or papillae, on your tongue; there are between one and more than a hundred per papilla.

Each of us has around 10,000 taste buds on average – women have more than men. Each one contains about 50 to 100 specialised receptor cells, each with a tiny hair that senses chemicals dissolved in saliva and transmits messages to the brain through various different nerves, depending on the location of the taste bud.

There's something special about taste and smell receptors – unlike most nerve cells, they can be replaced when they're old or damaged. In fact an average taste bud is renewed every 10 to 14 days. So why do some taste sensations tend to diminish with age? There is some evidence that the replacement process gets older too, and less efficient. But this does

a taste bud

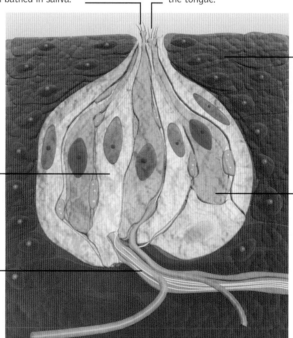

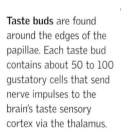

Gustatory hairs – these microvilli (tiny hairs) act as sensory receptors when bathed in saliva.

A pore, sometimes called a taste pore, on the surface of the tongue.

Taste buds are found around the edges of the papillae. Each taste bud contains about 50 to 100 gustatory cells that send nerve impulses to the brain's taste sensory cortex via the thalamus.

Epithelial cells make up the outermost layer – the epithelium – of the tongue.

Supporting cells separate the taste, or gustatory, cells from each other and from the epithelium.

Gustatory cells, also called taste cells, are the specialised receptor cells that transmit nerve impulses from the gustatory hairs to the nerve fibres.

Nerve fibres transmit impulses from the gustatory cells to the thalamus within the brain.

If your mouth burns after eating curry, drinking water won't help as the chemical in chillies is not water-soluble.

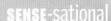

not explain why often only specific tastes are affected, rather than taste in general. Recent evidence suggests that in the elderly oral hygiene is also a significant factor.

TASTE IS EVERYWHERE

As well as the taste buds, there are taste receptors in most parts of your mouth, even extending down your throat. Babies have lots of them, but as they get older their sensitivity reduces and taste sensation comes predominantly from the tongue.

As children also have more working taste buds on the tongue, they taste things much more strongly than adults – which is one reason why children tend to dislike strong flavours, and our tastes 'mature' as we get older, so we may develop a liking for olives, beer, extra-strong mints, coffee or dark chocolate that we couldn't stand as children.

In addition to taste receptors, we also have nerve endings in both the mouth and nose (as we do on our skin) that detect hot, cold, strong or irritating substances – pepper, chilli, onions and ammonia, for example, as well as strong mint tastes and the effect of carbonation (fizzing) in drinks.

This is our so-called 'common chemical sense'. The nerve endings lie in the tongue surrounding the taste buds and transmit information to the brain down yet another separate nerve pathway, which also detects touch and texture sensations (important especially to the pleasure of eating foods with a high fat content). It's because there are multiple pathways transmitting such varieties of information to the brain that even when our sense of taste is impaired, our mouth can still sense the effects of food – such as its feel, or whether it is hot or cold.

SENSE-sational

THE PAIN AND THE PLEASURE OF CHILLI PEPPERS

If you eat hot spicy foods, such as chillies, you stimulate heat pain receptors in your mouth. Your brain interprets this as excess heat, often resulting in sweating and flushing in the head and neck area – known medically as 'gustatory sweating'. Frequent chilli eaters generally find the response reduces with time – but this is because chilli can desensitise the nerve endings, so they are reduce or 'switched off' and no longer respond (though after a respite, they will usually recover). If your mouth is burning, drinking a glass of water won't help because the chemical in chilli peppers is not water-soluble. Alcohol works better, so have a glass of wine or beer with your curry or, best of all, yoghurt – the fat content counteracts the chilli, which is why it's a good idea to order a yoghurt-based lassi or raita with a hot curry.

the emotional link

Have you ever found yourself transported back in time by a sudden whiff of a forgotten smell? You took your child into primary school for the first time, and suddenly images from your own schooldays flashed across your mind? Or you walk past someone wearing a particular scent and memories of your grandmother come flooding back?

And have you ever noticed particular aromas that can affect your feelings? Delight at the scent of new-mown grass, or sensations of unease whenever you smell a particular furniture polish, perhaps? It's because the area in the brain that first receives smell or taste impulses from the olfactory receptors or taste buds is one of its oldest and most primitive parts. Known as the limbic system, it also deals with emotions and emotional responses to memory. Only later is this information transmitted further to more recent areas of the brain involved with thinking, where smells and tastes are consciously perceived and interpreted.

That's why strong smells usually evoke strong responses – people either love them or hate them. Distinctive smells also leave lasting impressions that are closely linked to the memory of what was going on when you first smelled them. As the limbic system also controls mood, motivation, pain and pleasure sensations and some hormonal secretions, smells can have a powerful effect on our feelings. 'Smell is unique among the senses in its privileged access to the subconscious', says smell expert Professor Tim Jacob of Cardiff University.

SENSE-sational

THE SCENT OF DANGER

A keen nose will quickly detect smoke or a gas leak. Now scientists have shown that the human brain can sense even more subtle changes in smell, if the brain associates them with danger. In a study reported in the US journal *Science*, researchers exposed 12 volunteers to two 'grassy' odours and none could distinguish between them. Next, they administered a mild electric shock before the volunteers smelled one of the odours, and repeated the test. All volunteers could then distinguish one smell from the other, illustrating an ability which is 'evolutionary' says Dr Wen Li of the Feinberg School of Medicine, Northwestern University, Chicago. The research suggests that our distant ancestors developed an enhanced sense of smell to detect predators.

learning to smell

Whether we like or dislike smells is to some extent a learned response. Children are often less fussy about odours than adults, though even babies will respond with disgust to the smell of rotten food. As we mature, we

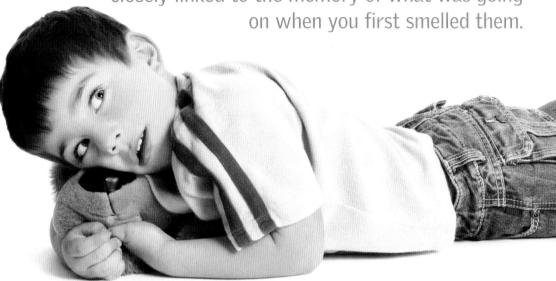

Distinctive smells also leave lasting impressions that are closely linked to the memory of what was going on when you first smelled them.

begin to develop odour preferences, which are influenced by familiarity. That explains, for instance, why urban dwellers who opt for country living may find livestock and manure smells unbearably offensive, while people who've grown up around farms accept them as perfectly normal.

Learned smell preferences also influence our food likes and dislikes. As you've discovered, much of the flavour of food is due to smell sensations. But, unlike taste, humans don't seem to have any innate preferences for particular food smells, other than a general distaste for the smell of rotting foodstuff.

Whether we like or dislike a particular flavour may thus depend as much on the circumstances in which we first encountered it as on its actual taste – but thereafter, if we associate a particular smell with something delicious to eat, it's likely to stimulate our appetite. On the other hand, learning is also how we develop an 'acquired taste' – repeated exposure to particular flavours tends to overcome original dislikes.

your smart sense plan

By now you probably know a lot more about taste and smell than most people, because these senses generally attract relatively little attention. And you also understand why they're important, and some of the 'enemies' that can damage or reduce them. In the next chapter you'll learn what steps you can take now to preserve and enhance these enjoyable senses, so you can both stay safe and continue to savour the flavours of life.

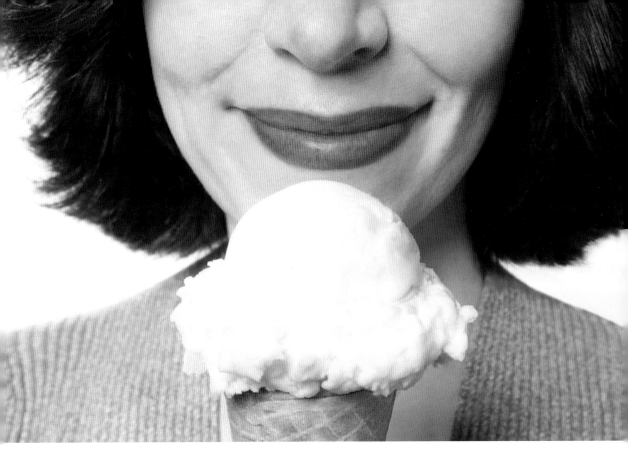

A keener sense
of taste and smell

13

What is really worrying about taste and smell is that – according to some scientists – as we get older we're beginning to lose these senses faster than perhaps any previous generation. This may sound frightening but it is just a warning. The good news is that this need not happen to you and this chapter will explain why.

We know that our senses of smell and taste – especially smell – tend to diminish with age. But why should people be losing their senses of taste and smell more quickly than they did in the past? The answers are key to your *Smart Sense Plan* because you can do something about it. This acceleration is not inevitable.

The book's introduction mentioned Dr Charles Spence, an experimental psychologist at Oxford University. In 2002 he wrote a fascinating report called 'Secrets of the Senses' in which he explained that, according to his department's research, there is every indication that, increasingly, we rely on sight to the detriment of other senses.

Dr Spence believes that because we now live in a visually dominant society – we are in danger of suffering from visual overload. In a fast-moving world, we look and react. Our eyes 'overdose on information', while our emotional senses, such as touch and smell, are neglected.

CRUNCHINESS

Curiously, another sense – hearing – also helps us to determine what we are eating, says experimental psychologist, Dr Charles Spence. 'The feel of food in your mouth is determined largely by the sound of it in your ear,' says Dr Spence. In an intriguing experiment to demonstrate this, he collaborated with renowned chef Heston Blumenthal at his Fat Duck restaurant in Bray, Berkshire. They asked diners to eat while wearing headphones that picked up the sound of the food being chewed, then played this back slightly altered – and found that, yes, it effectively changed people's perception of the crispness or crunchiness of their food.

Taste is also undoubtedly influenced by aroma, colour, texture and presentation ...

use it or lose it

Indulging ourselves, stimulating our non-visual senses for pure pleasure and savouring the effects, will keep them keen and make us healthier and happier, says Dr Spence. And the more senses you can stimulate simultaneously, the better it is for you. What's more, practising your sense skills will counter the deterioration of taste and smell that can cause the health and nutritional problems in later life, mentioned earlier.

Take one simple experience – drinking a glass of wine. For true wine-lovers, the experience and the pleasure isn't just about taste (or the effects of alcohol), it's about the depth of colour, temperature, fragrance and feel in your mouth. For taste is undoubtedly influenced by aroma, colour, texture and presentation – as well as all the flavours you will be able to detect as you train your taste buds to be more perceptive.

FOCUS ON YOUR FOOD

Protect is the first step in your **PACE** strategy and, interestingly, one way you can do this is by paying more attention to what you're tasting or smelling. Psychologists know that the more you focus on any particular

Continued on p196 ▶

super-tasters

When it comes to experiencing taste, people are not all created equal. Some people are natural 'super-tasters' because they are born with more taste buds than others, so are better able to distinguish different flavours and react more strongly to different foods.

Women lead the field. According to research at Yale University in the USA, about 35 per cent of women – but only 15 per cent of men – are such 'super-tasters'. It is also thought that there are genetic variations – with Asians and Africans more likely to be super-tasters than people from other ethnic backgrounds. Super-tasters experience all taste sensations more intensely, especially bitter or sweet tastes.

Among individuals of European descent, it is estimated that about 25 per cent of the population are super-tasters and around half are 'normal' tasters. The other 25 per cent are often described as non-tasters, although low-tasters would be a more accurate term, as they can perceive tastes, but not so well. For this group, the experience of food is less intense than normal, and they are relatively insensitive to bitter tastes. These are the people who will happily 'eat anything', and are usually not particularly fussy about how their food is prepared.

. . . 25 per cent of the population are super-tasters and around half are 'normal' tasters. The other 25 per cent are often described as non-tasters.

NEON TASTES

On taste scales, super-tasters seem to perceive sweetness or bitterness roughly three times as intensely as other people. 'Super-tasters live in a neon taste world, and non-tasters live in a pastel taste world', says Professor Linda M. Bartoshuk, who heads the Yale research team and coined the term.

Not surprisingly then, super-tasters tend to be fussy eaters with strong likes and dislikes – they often loathe foods and drinks with distinctive bitter flavours such as coffee, beer, grapefruit, cabbage, Brussels sprouts and spinach. They generally find sugary foods sickeningly sweet, and are highly sensitive to the fat content of food – they can often instantly distinguish semi-skimmed from skimmed milk, for example. And, as super-tasters also have more sensation nerve-endings in their tongues, they tend to find the burning sensation more intense when they eat 'hot' foods such as chilli peppers.

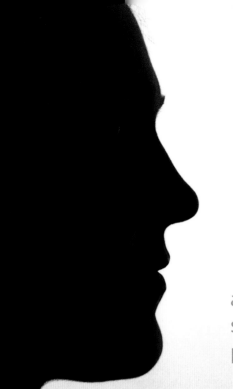

Super-tasters have a big advantage in certain careers, such as being a chef or a professional wine-taster.

THE GENETIC LINK

Scientists studying these variations in taste sensitivity have found that they are linked with variations in the size and distribution of the papillae on the tongue, the tiny bumps containing the taste buds. Normal or medium tasters have an average number of medium-sized papillae. Super-tasters have more papillae, and these are smaller and more closely packed together, whereas non-tasters have fewer papillae, which are larger and more widely spaced.

The phenomenon of super-tasters seems to be based on genetic differences – people with a particular genetic make-up can taste a chemical called 6-n-propylthiouracil, PROP for short, while others cannot. This formed the basis for the Yale University tests. If volunteers are asked to chew on a piece of paper impregnated with PROP, super-tasters generally find it extremely unpleasant, and many spit it out because it tastes so bitter. Non-tasters and medium tasters just taste paper.

Discovering your own taster status will help you to understand your own food preferences and those of others. If you've ever wondered why someone is so faddy or always seems to ask for something different, this may be the reason. One person's picky eating is another's discriminating palate – so super-tasters have a big advantage in certain careers, such as being a chef or a professional wine-taster.

SENSE-sational

£10 MILLION TASTE BUDS

Wine expert and TV presenter Angela Mount is one of a select band of wine buyers who have been widely credited with revolutionising the British attitude to wine, and introducing quality wine to high street shoppers. Her former employers, Somerfield supermarkets, thought so highly of her abilities that, in 2003, they insured her taste buds for £10 million.

sensation, the stronger it seems. So be aware when you eat: think about the taste, the smell and the sound of your food, how it feels in your mouth, its texture and temperature and spiciness. Savour every mouthful. And concentrate on the experience; don't read or watch TV while you eat.

The presentation of food is important, too, as you will discover later when we offer some tips for boosting sensations. It is also helpful to expand your awareness of tastes, exercising this sense as much as you can – eat a wide variety of foods, and try some new ones, experiment with different combinations or ways of cooking, or add spices and herbs that you don't usually use.

fad or super-sense?

It is easy to see how disharmony can occur when family members don't share the same tastes. What seems like little Johnny's wilful refusal to eat his broccoli or grapefruit could be due to his super-taster status – though, since this status is a genetic trait, at least one of his parents will have it too. Or he could be more taste-sensitive simply because of his age. If he is a genuine super-taster, it will be hard to convince him to like Brussels sprouts – though he may well grow to enjoy them as an adult. Suspect a super-taster if a child adamantly refuses bitter vegetables but also isn't especially fond of sweets.

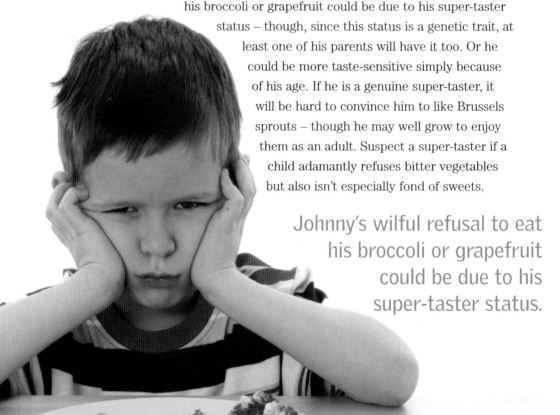

Johnny's wilful refusal to eat his broccoli or grapefruit could be due to his super-taster status.

practical performance test
How well do you taste?

Knowing your taster status could help you to assess how much you need to stimulate your taste sensations, and the best foods to choose – or avoid. It can also give important clues to other health risks. The Yale University team used a prescription-only drug in their research on super-tasters. But here's a simple test you can do at home, based on their experiments. You will need:

- a thick piece of paper and a hole punch or a paper-reinforcement ring
- a cotton bud
- blue food colouring
- a magnifying glass.

Punch a 7mm diameter hole in the paper and cut the paper around it so that it measures about 2cm square. Alternatively, and this is easier if you have one, use a paper-reinforcement ring – the sort you stick around hole-punched paper to prevent the hole tearing in a ring binder. Dip the cotton bud into the food colouring and swab it onto the tip of your tongue.

Place the paper with a hole in it or the reinforcement ring over the coloured area. You will see that the tongue has gone blue but has pink spots – these are the papillae that contain the taste buds, which do not take up the dye in food colouring. Use the magnifying glass to count the number of pink spots within the paper hole.

If you have between 15 and 35 pink spots you are a normal taster – like around half of the population. Fewer than 15 spots and you join the one in four people classed as non-tasters, whereas more than 35 and you are in the other quarter of the population who qualify as super-tasters. Who knows, if you are, maybe a new career as a wine-taster – or a chocolate-tester, if you prefer – could open up.

health impact

Interestingly, knowing your taster status could help you to protect your good health – or at least make you cautious. For instance, it seems that people who do not have an acute sense of taste are more likely to drink or smoke. By contrast, some studies have shown that super-tasters tend to drink less alcohol because alcohol activates bitter taste receptors and, for the same reason, are less likely to smoke.

As they tend to avoid high-fat and sugary foods, super-tasters may also be less likely to become overweight. Further research at Yale has suggested that among older women, those who are super-tasters tend to be thinner and weigh less than average, with a lower percentage of body fat. They also had more HDL-cholesterol, the 'good' fat in the bloodstream, and fewer 'bad' triglycerides – which may explain why they also tend to have lower rates of cardiovascular disease.

Other research suggests, however, that male super-tasters sometimes behave differently. Instead of avoiding high-fat foods, they experience the extra taste sensation of fatty foods as pleasurable – and are thus more likely to gain weight.

Another disadvantage for super-tasters is that their taste buds may lead them to reject all the bitter-but-good-for-you vegetables – making them more vulnerable to certain diseases, including cancer. Researchers at Wayne State University, together with Professor Bartoshuk and colleagues at Yale, studied a group of older men undergoing colonoscopy, an examination of the lower bowel, and found that the super-taster members of the group had more colon polyps than the others. Polyps in the colon are a known risk factor for colon cancer. As further evidence, the men with more polyps had a lower vegetable intake and higher body weight – both also risk factors for colon cancer.

taste and personality

Your taster status may also affect your personality. Researchers from the Taste Science Laboratory at Cornell University in the USA have shown that decision-making strategies vary between 'non-tasters', who tend to rely more on logical reasoning, normal tasters, who tend to play things by ear and improvise, and super-tasters, who are more likely to mull things over and 'sleep' on complex problems.

This, they suggest, is because all types of taste and smell sensations are processed in the same area of the brain that considers contingencies and weighs values – so more stimulation in this area will prompt more of that type of decision making. The logical areas of the brain will dominate in those with less such sensory stimulation.

Finally, while we cannot change our taster status because it's all a question of genes, we can enhance our ability to taste through practice, by experimenting and widening our experience of different tastes, and even by staying cheerful and positive

SENSEalert

GO EASY WITH THE SALT

When people's taste is not so good, they often compensate by adding extra salt to their food. Not only is this a risk factor for high blood pressure, but also sensitivity to salty flavours reduces faster with age than other basic tastes. Older people tend to use two or three times as much salt on their food as younger individuals, and those taking medications that dull smell sensitivity may use as much as 12 times more salt. And it's easy not to appreciate just how much you are adding. So tip a small quantity of salt onto the side of your plate rather than sprinkling it all over, and try the suggestions for healthier alternatives on the page opposite.

(as you'll discover in the next chapter), as negative moods such as anxiety and depression can affect tasting ability.

enhance the pleasure

How many times have you heard someone say that a particular food doesn't taste the way it did when they were young? Perhaps you have said it yourself. Part of this may indeed be due to changes in farming or production methods, but some of it could be a result of reduced taste or smell sensations as people get older.

It's important not to allow this to stop you eating – and enjoying – a balanced diet. Altering ingredients and varying the way you prepare, present and season foods can make a big difference. And as we've seen, enlarging the range of your smell and taste experiences can help to preserve these gratifying senses.

ALTERNATIVES TO SALT

Try using stronger flavours and more herbs and spices to compensate for reduced taste and smell, or just to enhance your sensory experiences. For extra flavour, look at the list of umami-rich foods on page 187 – including mushrooms, ripe tomatoes and ginger; any of these can add an extra tang to a meal. It doesn't have to be complicated: you can create the taste with simple ingredients such as grated Parmesan cheese, or Worcestershire, soy or Thai fish sauce – all high in natural glutamates. Just a dash of ketchup can work wonders.

Even people who have no sense of smell, a condition called anosmia, usually still retain some basic taste sensations from their tongue and mouth. Adding pepper or other spices to food stimulates the nerve endings of the common chemical sense, (see page 189) and this can help in distinguishing other tastes.

SENSE-sational

CURRIES SET YOUR PULSE RACING

People get more from a curry than just its spicy taste, according to scientists at Nottingham Trent University. They discovered that the combination of tastes in a curry stimulate far more taste receptors (and heat pain receptors) than traditional British meals such as fish and chips – and the effect raises your heart rate. Chicken korma increased the heart rate of their study participants by an average three beats per minute, tikka masala by four and a half, and rogan josh by seven. Fish and chips did virtually nothing.

In this way, curries arouse the senses and provide a 'natural high'. Lead researcher Professor Stephen Gray comments: 'By activating several areas of the tongue simultaneously, we are dazzling our taste buds.' Just remember, though, that curries with creamy sauces tend to be high in fat and calories as well.

Or try monosodium glutamate (MSG) itself, the glutamate seasoning described on page 187. If you live in the UK you'll probably have to visit a Chinese supermarket to find it, or you could buy it online (try under the Oriental name Aji-No-Moto). In the USA or Asia, it's more readily available from ordinary grocery stores – in many parts of Asia, cooks add a dash of MSG just as we might add salt or sugar.

Despite its bad press, MSG is simply concentrated glutamate – the same substance found naturally in foods and produced in all our bodies – which is then stabilised with salt. But MSG contains only a third of the amount of sodium in table salt, so using it instead can reduce your salt intake. Plus, you don't need much – add around half a teaspoon to 500g of meat or to season four to six servings of vegetables. Most scientists now say there's no evidence to support health concerns.

Other concentrated food essences, extracts, bouillons or stock cubes can easily be used to enhance flavour when cooking rice or pasta, for instance. Or experiment with the vast choice of culinary herbs now readily available to stimulate your taste with more and varied sensations.

THINK ABOUT PRESENTATION

The setting can make a big difference to your enjoyment of food. So lay the table attractively and add pretty garnishes to your meals. Go for colourful foods and attractive combinations, or add a side-salad or some fancy bread. Try to make meals sociable – chat, take your time, savour every bite. If you live alone, invite a friend or neighbour over for a meal occasionally – you could even test out new recipes on each other.

collect smell memories

In the same way that you have the ability to enhance your sense of taste, you can also improve your sense of smell and help to preserve it in good condition well into older age.

'Everyone can increase their olfactory ability by simply paying attention to scents,' says Dr Rachel Herz, a research psychologist at Brown University in Rhode Island in the USA, who has written a book on smell. Consciously noticing the smells around you can actually improve your sense of smell, she adds. And she recommends deliberately increasing the range of different smells that you are exposed to, especially those with emotional resonance – for example, by collecting scent mementos that evoke memories of special times, such as the soap from the hotel where you spent your honeymoon, or by cooking aromatic comfort food that your mother used to make.

YOUR SMELL-MEMORY BANK

Other evidence proves that your experience of one smell enhances your ability to identify other smells. Neurologists at Northwestern University in the USA have shown that after smelling a floral scent for a few minutes, people get better at identifying a variety of different floral smells. The same thing happened with those who experienced minty,

Human bloodhounds? With practice, people's sense of smell can become so acute that they can follow a scent-track just like a dog.

alcohol-based, or ketone-based smells (the chemical smell, like pear drops or nail varnish) – they became experts on other smells in those categories.

Brain scans also revealed that these smell experiences enhanced responses in the olfactory (smelling) areas of the brain in a way that reflected learning. The researchers say that learning to distinguish between similar smells like this enhances our ability to

HUMAN BLOODHOUNDS?

In one unusual experiment at the University of California, 32 student volunteers were persuaded to put on overalls, a blindfold, earplugs and gloves (to eliminate all clues from other senses), then get down on all fours and attempt to sniff out a 10m (33ft) chocolate trail laid through the grass on the university campus. Two-thirds of them managed to follow the trail to the end within three attempts, zigzagging along its path with their noses in the same way that dogs do.

The experiment was designed to discover if two nostrils are better than one (and yes, they are), but also revealed how training enhanced smell sensitivity. When four volunteers had more practice, they deviated less from the trail and nearly doubled their speed. 'If people practise sniffing smells, they can get really good at it', said lead researcher Jess Porter. 'Our sense of smell is less keen partly because we put less demand on it.'

Continued on p204 ▶

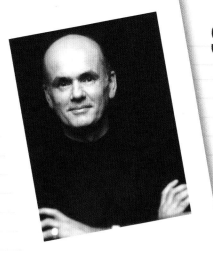

scents
and sensibility

Roja Dove

'**N**oses', in the world of fragrance, are the few experts who can recognise and distinguish between hundreds of different aromas. The skill is both innate and also honed over years of training, says Roja Dove, an internationally-renowned perfumer and leading authority on all aspects of the industry.

The smells of his childhood were the scent of woodland near his grandparents' Kent home, picking bluebells or the spicy aroma of his mother's baking as he lay in bed at night. 'When I look at my olfactive palate, I know they have all these things in them – earthy, woody, spicy – without question a product of my childhood.'

He rediscovered his earliest smell memory by chance when he sampled scents by Thierry Mugler inspired by the film 'Perfume'. 'They gave me one and I said "This reminds me of chewing leather!". It suddenly came back to me – not a smell but a taste, the two are so interlinked. As a toddler, I used to chew my leather reins and the taste and scent of wet leather was what I remembered.'

'When I look at my olfactive palate, I know they have all these things in them – earthy, woody, spicy – without question a product of my childhood.'

As a teenager, Roja became increasingly fascinated with perfumes and the world of perfumery, taking an especial interest in Guerlain. Its history became a passion – exquisitely rewarded when one enquiry elicited a bottle of Guerlain fragrance ('I think it was Habit Rouge'), a beautiful book and a vintage bottle. 'It was like Christmas collided with Nirvana!'

Persistence paid off when he was invited to join the company and began his perfumer's training. 'You're given, say, ten different raw materials to smell as oils, and commit to memory. You have a book which will sit with you for a lifetime in which you notate the association – it could be your grandmother's house, or a damp cellar. It's a memory game. You fill this book with olfactive associations. The next day you're given ten more, and that's how it builds up. You would normally stop at 40 to 50, then start comparing the oils to each other. So you first understand the oil on a personal level and then you start to learn it in a much more objective way and discover its olfactive qualities.

'There's a palette of around 3,000 raw materials – nobody would know all of them – but I would know several hundred.' Among them is the exclusive Jasmine de Grasse – at £28,000 a kilo, it is more expensive than gold bullion and only used by him, Guerlain, Chanel and Jean Patou. 'I'm the only private individual who buys it', he says.

'When I create a perfume, I use around 80 per cent natural material; the industry average today is 15 to 20 per cent.' Overly synthetic modern scents upset him – 'they don't breathe, these monolithic structures'.

'And if I'm making a bespoke scent, I normally ask clients if they would avoid drinking coffee and alcohol or eating spiced food for 24 hours,' he says. 'It comes through the skin and on the breath.'

When working, he prefers the odours around him to be neutral, which is why, in his opulent Haute Parfumerie at Harrods – all black lacquer, crystal chandeliers and Lalique glass – you smell nothing until a bottle is opened and its fragrance released.

'And if I'm making a bespoke scent, I normally ask clients if they would avoid drinking coffee and alcohol or eating spiced food for 24 hours,' he says. 'It comes through the skin and on the breath.'

His own diet is 'incredibly healthy', he adds – fish, plenty of fresh fruit and vegetables, lots of water, no meat and no fried or fatty foods. 'But I'm not a fanatic about anything. Life for me is about balance. It's built-in self-protection.'

It pays dividends. He rarely has a cold but, if he does, the loss of smell is acute. 'I feel totally claustrophobic, as if I'm blind to the world and the world has gone silent.'

It saddens him that so few people value a sense that can bring so much enjoyment. 'I tell people "Stop! Just stop!" I was walking past the Ritz the other day and I suddenly smelled jasmine; it was planted in the window boxes. It was wonderful! But most people are so busy rushing around that they would never have noticed it.

'People rarely stop to think about their sense of smell but it is a crucial, vital sense. How each of us respond to odour is totally personal – I call it our olfactory fingerprint, because it is as unique as a fingerprint.

'The key to enhancing this sense is to indulge it and cultivate it. Buy a small quantity of different essential oils and pour a little into your bathwater. Buy neroli, it induces a sense of well-being. Explore the smells around you and create a private "carnet de voyage", a little book where you write what you discover. That's the true magic of scent. It transports us in an instant to mothers and lovers and places we've visited. It's profound.'

A ROSE BY ANY OTHER NAME...

... might not smell as sweet after all. Researchers at Oxford University offered a group of people a smell rather like Brie (a soft cheese) and asked them to rate the aroma. For some of them it was labelled 'Cheddar cheese', while others were informed it was 'body odour'. Those who were told they were smelling cheese rated the scent as more pleasant. Perhaps Shakespeare didn't get this one quite right.

appreciate the immense richness of aromas in everyday life. Our past experiences – so-called learnt responses – may also explain why our expectations play a role in smell perceptions.

Pleasant aromas can make us feel more positive. People also respond – to a lesser extent – to placebo fragrances: those exposed to an odourless substance but told that it's something nice often report feeling better.

And we may link particular smells with information from other senses, for example, people are more likely to identify a smell, such as that of cherries or strawberries, if they're looking at something red at the same time. Again, you can use this information to enhance your taste and smell, for example by making sure you appreciate all the sensory aspects of eating – the colour, presentation, texture, flavour and aroma – or by gazing at a flower and touching the petals as you smell it.

Exercising your sense of smell – using it frequently and consciously – undoubtedly enhances it.

Exercising your sense of smell – using it frequently and consciously – undoubtedly enhances it. Those who perform best in smell identification tests are people who have honed their skills. Frequent practice makes such a difference that smell scientists have difficulty undertaking research, because volunteers tend to perform better the more they participate.

BE SNIFFY ABOUT IT

You may also find that it helps to sniff more – despite the dictates of good manners. According to research at the University of Pennsylvania, published in 2007, the olfactory receptors in the roof of our noses respond to mechanical pressure (such as physical sniffing) as well as odour molecules, and send messages to the brain in exactly the same way.

This explains why we sniff to smell something, and why our sense of smell is synchronised with inhaling, something that previously had been a mystery despite 50 years of research. So sniffing enhances the sensitivity of the nose and boosts our ability to smell, especially to detect weaker odours.

safeguard your senses

Being aware of your senses of taste and smell and consciously using and enjoying them will undoubtedly help you to preserve them. And, as you read in the last chapter, there are many other preventable or treatable conditions that can affect them. The following chapters will tell you more about smell and taste disorders and what your doctor may be able to do to help. Here are some steps you can take to avoid other possible reasons for reduced smell or taste sensation.

Don't smoke As explained earlier in the book, it can damage your eyesight and, unsurprisingly, the tar and smoke is also likely to affect your taste and smell senses. See your GP or look at our Resources section (page 238) for help with quitting.

Protect your head Head injuries are a common cause of loss of taste and smell. While some accidents are unavoidable, there are sensible precautions. Always wear a properly-fitting helmet on a bicycle or motorbike, and for activities such as horse-riding or ice-skating. Make sure your car seat belts are securely anchored and fit properly, and always 'belt up'.

Wash your hands Colds and other respiratory infections impair your taste and smell while you have them, and occasionally cause lasting damage. It's a rare outcome from any one cold, but because respiratory infections are so

Protect your head – head injuries are a common cause of loss of taste and smell.

common, their after-effects are a leading cause of loss of taste and smell, especially among older people. So it is sensible to steer clear of anyone with an obvious sniffle (and stay at home if you are affected), but you can do much more than that.

Research has shown repeatedly that hand-washing significantly reduces your chance of catching a cold. If hand-washing is difficult or inconvenient, keep a little bottle of hand sanitiser gel in your pocket or bag. You are four times more likely to pick up someone's cold from hand-to-hand contact than from a sneeze. Viruses can survive for hours on hard surfaces such as telephones or door knobs.

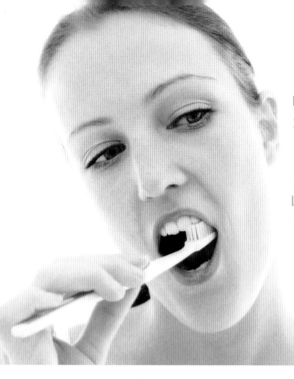

Eat good food Reduced smell and taste as you get older can affect appetite and lead to nutritional deficiencies that may impair taste and smell senses. Eat a healthy, balanced diet to avoid this vicious circle.

Look after your teeth Dental disease, mouth infections and poor oral hygiene can impair both appetite and taste sensations. Make sure you clean your teeth at least twice daily and go for regular dental check-ups. Tongue cleaning is also important; in studies, it has been shown to greatly improve taste, particularly in the elderly.

Dental disease, mouth infections and poor oral hygiene can impair both appetite and taste sensations. Make sure you clean your teeth properly at least twice daily.

Avoid nasty smells Some foul odours may impair your ability to smell. Culprits include certain moulds, industrial chemicals, petroleum products and cleaning solutions. If you are exposed for a long time or on a regular basis, wear a mask impregnated with odour-reducing compounds to cover your nose and mouth while working with them. At work an employer should provide such masks (sometimes described as 'nuisance odour respirators'). For personal protection from DIY products or household chemicals, look for a carbon/charcoal filter such as the Carbosorb Plus Facemask from www.conservation-by-design.co.uk

BOOST YOUR SENSES

Although relatively little research has been done to identify specific dietary ingredients or supplements that might enhance taste or smell, some supplements may help in certain cases.

● **Zinc** This mineral is most often recommended to enhance both smell and taste, since it is known to be involved in the smell signalling responses of olfactory receptors. Zinc tends to be depleted when you have respiratory infections, but the link with impaired smell has not been proved. There is also some evidence that a reduced sensitivity to smell caused by a poor diet may be due in part to low zinc levels. Many people on Western diets are relatively zinc deficient, so it makes sense to try to ensure an adequate intake. Good food sources include red meat, poultry, beans, lentils, nuts (especially pecan nuts), sunflower and pumpkin seeds, and whole grains. Zinc supplements are sometimes used to treat smell and taste disorders, but again there is no conclusive evidence that they are effective. The recommended dose is usually 25mg to 30mg daily.

● Vitamin E According to a study at the Taste and Smell Clinic in Washington, DC, low vitamin E levels may be linked with reduced smell and taste. Researchers assessed 250 patients with taste and smell dysfunctions and found that their average vitamin E intake was just 36 per cent of the recommended daily allowance – significantly below adequate levels. It's not clear what role vitamin E plays, but it may be important for renewal of both taste and olfactory receptors. Vitamin E is found in leafy green vegetables, broccoli and soya beans; it's best to boost your food intake rather than taking supplements.

● Alpha-lipoic acid Preliminary results of a small study at the University of Dresden Medical School in Germany have suggested that alpha-lipoic acid, an antioxidant that helps maintain nerve cell function, may improve loss of smell following respiratory infections. Twenty-three patients with either diminished or no smell sensation took 600mg of alpha-lipoic acid a day for an average of 4.5 months, and 60 per cent showed a significant improvement on olfactory tests. But the researchers caution that further studies are needed as spontaneous recovery can occur in such cases up to two years after the infection.

indulge your senses

You are now probably more aware of your senses of taste and smell and the role they play. You're armed with some excellent strategies to Protect these senses, and the fact that practice can actually improve them. You've learnt how to Assess and test your taster status – which is fun, interesting and could also help you to avoid certain health problems. So you've taken two steps in your PACE strategy for better taste and smell. But, with these senses, the key is enjoyment. According to Dr Spence, the experimental psychologist from Oxford University mentioned earlier, we should all seek to indulge these and our other senses a little more – to fulfil our basic need for a balanced multi-sensory diet, as boosting all our senses will make us more productive and successful, and also enhance our relationships.

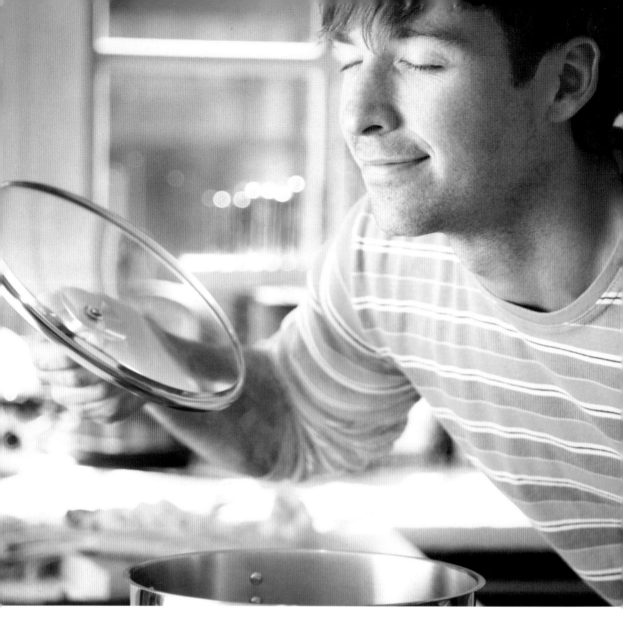

Check and assess

14

The good news for everyone who enjoys good food and delights in everyday scents and aromas is that, unlike other nerve cells, taste and smell receptors are replaced throughout our lives.

But, because they are replaced more slowly as we get older, our senses of smell and taste tend to become blunted to some degree, although there is a great deal that we can do to compensate and preserve them.

One important reason why you should never accept deterioration in your smell and taste as just another consequence of ageing is that sometimes taste and smell disorders signal other conditions, many of which can be treated. In fact, some scientific studies have suggested that ageing itself is less responsible for the decreases in these senses than the accumulation of other bodily conditions and environmental influences over the decades. And, if the condition causing the loss of sensations is treated, taste and smell sensitivity will often recover.

This chapter explains some reasons why your taste and smell senses may become weaker. And you'll learn some quick and simple ways to assess the senses yourself because generally they fade slowly and it's easy not to notice. (Remember, Assess is the second stage of your **PACE** plan.)

WHAT HAPPENS WITH AGE?

Although the body constantly replaces taste buds, the rate of replacement tends to slow down in middle age, slightly faster in women than in men, and the buds themselves become smaller. Taste sense rarely falls off significantly until after the age of 60 though, and even then most people retain reasonable sensitivity. If taste sensation is lost, it's usually bitter and sour tastes that last longest, presumably as a protective mechanism.

practical performance test
Taste the difference

You can test your sensitivity for sweet, sour, bitter and salt tastes quite simply. Make up the following solutions in separate jars or shallow dishes, being careful to use different spoons for each one:

- ½ teaspoon table sugar dissolved in 2 tablespoons water (sweet)
- ½ teaspoon lemon juice dissolved in 2 tablespoons water (sour)
- 2 tablespoons black coffee, allowed to cool, or tonic water (bitter)
- ⅛ teaspoon table salt dissolved in 2 tablespoons water (salty)

Ideally, ask someone else to drizzle a couple of drops of each solution onto your tongue while you close your eyes. If there's no one else around, you'll have to promise yourself not to cheat Rinse your mouth well with water between each test sample. You should be able to name each taste and to experience it as quite different to any of the others. If not, talk to your GP.

As it's difficult to get hold of MSG in this country (except as soy sauce, which is quite salty), the easiest way to test your umami taste receptors is to check that you can still taste a favourite food by placing a small sliver of something like cooked mushroom on your tongue (see page 187 for a more complete list). Again, if you can't tell what it is, talk to your GP.

smell check

Our smell sense is rather more likely to become impaired as we get older. In fact, some tests suggest that our smelling ability peaks at around the age of eight, and begins to decline from as early as 15. In practical terms though, it's usually only after the age of 60 that there's any noticeable deterioration in smelling capacity.

practical performance test
How well can you smell?

To take the alcohol sniff test (AST) – a basic smell function test developed at the University of California San Diego Nasal Dysfunction Clinic – you will need alcohol wipes (available from pharmacies), the little disposable pads that doctors use to sterilise the skin before taking blood or giving injections. You can test yourself but it's easier with the help of a partner or friend.

- Tear the top off the packet so that around a third to a half of the pad is exposed. The person taking the test should take an initial sniff, so that they recognise the smell.
- The tester now holds the pad away and asks the subject to close their eyes and breathe normally – this is important, as deep breathing or deliberate sniffing will invalidate the results. The pad is then held at the subject's mid-chest height and very slowly moved vertically upwards towards the nose, about 1cm closer every time the person breathes out. At the point where the person first says he or she can detect the alcohol smell, measure the distance from the bottom of the nose to the pad. It should be 20cm or more.
- If you're not sure, repeat the test two or three times to check that the results are consistent. If the distance is less than 20cm, or the subject cannot smell the pad at all, he or she should probably consult a GP, as more specialist tests will help to pinpoint the problem. (The AST is not a perfect test because alcohol also stimulates the nerve endings of the common chemical sense that responds to pain and irritants, so even people with smell loss might be able to detect it.)

taste loss is rare

Most people who experience loss of taste sensations – ageusia – in fact have a problem with smelling, as mentioned earlier. Taste disorders are rare and often there is no obvious cause. Frequently, the sense recovers by itself, though it may take months or years. Head injury or some rare diseases can cause taste loss and, strangely, people with diabetes may lose their taste sensitivity yet retain normal smelling capacity.

If you notice a metallic taste especially when eating, using plastic rather than metal cutlery can help.

Most of those affected have diminished taste rather than complete loss – taste sensations may be blunted, or it may be difficult to distinguish between tastes. It's also possible for taste disorders to feature spontaneous taste sensations, which may sometimes be unpleasant. Some people complain of a metallic taste in their mouth. Simple solutions for bad tastes are to chew gum or suck on mints. If you notice a metallic taste especially when eating, using plastic rather than metal cutlery can help.

Dental or oral hygiene problems As mentioned in the last chapter, various dental problems can interfere with taste sensations – and sometimes with smell as well – so if you have painful or ill-fitting dentures, gum disease or tooth decay, consult your dentist. Cleaning your tongue can also help; use a toothbrush or a special plastic tongue scraper, available from pharmacies.

Dry mouth Another potentially treatable problem that may affect your sense of taste is a dry mouth. To detect its taste, food needs to be dissolved. As saliva flow diminishes with age, this may be a problem. Suspect dry mouth if you also find swallowing difficult or uncomfortable – and do mention it to your GP as there are many other possible causes.

Dry mouth can also be associated with diabetes and certain auto-immune disorders, such as Sjögren's syndrome, which destroys moisture-producing glands. Or sometimes salivary glands have been blocked or damaged by disease, radiation or surgery. Dry mouth can be a side effect of some medicines, including antidepressants and antihistamines. Your GP may be able to change your medication and resolve the problem very simply, or prescribe a drug to boost saliva flow.

GET THE JUICES FLOWING

● Ask your pharmacist about artificial saliva products. Like the artificial tears mentioned in chapter 4, you can buy these over-the-counter – and indeed, dry mouth and dry eyes sometimes occur simultaneously.

SENSEalert

BITTER BLOOD PRESSURE PILLS

If you're taking medication for high blood pressure and notice odd changes in your taste sensations, check which drug you're on. A strongly metallic, bitter or even sweet taste in your mouth may be a side effect of a class of drugs called angiotensin-converting enzyme (ACE) inhibitors, especially a medicine called captopril (Capoten). If you're affected, ask your GP if it is possible to change your tablets to something else.

---

practical performance test
What does it taste like?

The basic sniff test on page 210 tests your orthonasal smelling capacity – the ability to detect smells outside the body. Here's a simple check of your retronasal sensation – the internal smelling mechanism that helps you to taste food. Take a small cube of peeled apple and a cube of raw peeled potato cut to the same size. Put them in two identical containers and move them around so you don't know which is which (or ask someone else to do this for you). Then, with your eyes closed and your nose firmly pinched, lick or nibble each cube in turn. Most people can't tell the difference. That's because apple and potato are virtually indistinguishable by taste alone. Let go of your nose and try again, and you'll usually have no trouble telling them apart.

- Take care with mouthwashes – some contain alcohol or peroxide that dry out your mouth even more. Ask your dentist about toothpastes and mouthwashes that are specially formulated for people with dry mouth.
- Keep up your water intake – take frequent sips throughout the day and keep a glass by your bed at night.
- Avoid alcohol, which has a drying effect in the mouth and causes dehydration that will make dry mouth worse.
- Avoid tea, coffee, colas, cocoa and hot chocolate for the same reason, and cut back on acidic foods and drinks, such as citrus fruit or juices.
- Cut down on salt – it will make your dry mouth worse – and avoid very dry or high salt foods, such as crisps or crackers.
- Chew gum or suck boiled sweets to boost saliva flow.

SMELL AFFECTS TASTE

Losing your sense of smell, known medically as anosmia, is much more common than pure loss of taste. But this can affect your taste, too, because the two senses are so closely linked.

Around half of people aged 65 to 80 and about three-quarters of those over 80 have some loss of smell, probably due to loss of smell receptors or nerve endings in the nose. Yet, some 80-year-olds perform on smell tests just as well as young adults. Women often fare better than men – at all ages they tend to have greater sensitivity to smell.

Because taste bud cells can be replaced, even in old age, people with complete anosmia can usually still distinguish salty, sweet, bitter and sour tastes on the tongue. The problem is usually distinguishing between more subtle tastes – which can affect enjoyment of food – and could be one reason that older people may complain that foods do not taste as good as they once did.

the smell of sadness

Not surprisingly perhaps, people who lose their sensations of smell and taste may become depressed. But the link seems to work the other way round, too – depressed people have reduced taste and smell sensitivity.

The relationship is complex. For instance, it's hard to know which comes first, as most depressed people have not been tested for sensory disorders before the onset of their illness, and people with sensory disorders are not routinely checked for depression.

Researchers at Tel Aviv University in Israel studied a group of women and found that those who were depressed also tended to lose their sense of smell. The same researchers also considered the effects of auto-immune disorders such as lupus and rheumatoid arthritis in which auto-antibodies attack the body's own tissues. They believe that the auto-antibodies weaken smell sensitivity and provoke depression, explaining why these symptoms are so common among those affected.

taste test

Scientists at Bristol University in the UK have also found key chemical changes linked with both depression and taste. Depression is associated with reductions in two brain chemicals called serotonin and noradrenaline. As these are also present in taste buds, the researchers reasoned that they could also affect taste sensitivity.

thinkSENSE ● ● ●

WARNING SIGNS

If you do experience a loss of smell or taste sensations, watch out for symptoms of depression – they can creep up without you being aware of them and seriously interfere with work, social and family life. Symptoms can be physical as well as emotional. Classic signs include loss of appetite, indigestion, constipation or diarrhoea, unexplained aches and pains and, especially, waking up regularly in the early hours of the morning and being unable to get back to sleep. As antidepressants may help both conditions, do talk to your GP if you experience a loss of smell or taste and you feel miserable.

They gave volunteers different antidepressant drugs that raise levels of one or other of these chemicals, and found that increased serotonin levels also improved sensitivity to sweet and bitter tastes, while increased noradrenaline levels improved sensitivity to bitter and sour tastes. A placebo (dummy) drug had no effect on taste sensations.

This raises the possibility of using a taste test not just to diagnose depression, but also to work out which brain chemical is affected and so determine which drug might work best in treatment.

Continued on p216 ▶

take care!

Taste and smell are the two senses that actively encourage us to eat – making them key tools in the human survival kit. When they're lost – to any degree – some people become much less interested in food and may forget or skip meals. Others use too much salt.

Losing interest in food is especially worrying when someone already has a poor appetite, because of illness, perhaps, as they are then at risk of nutritional deficiency. Equally dangerous is the tendency of others, who opt for more strongly flavoured, fried, high-fat, high-salt processed foods that pile on the calories and weight, endangering their health in other ways.

SENSIBLE PRECAUTIONS

But our senses of taste and smell are not only important for nourishment. They are also an early warning system. People who cannot smell may fail to detect a gas leak or a chip-pan fire. They may not realise that a piece of fish smells rank – leaving them vulnerable to food poisoning. In one study, nearly three-quarters of patients with anosmia had experienced some difficulties with cooking, and half reported having accidentally eaten rotten food.

If you live with someone else who has full smell capacity, this may not be such a problem. If you live alone and cook for yourself, be extra careful – always check and abide by cooking times and use-by dates. Throw away food that is past the recommended storage time, or has been left unrefrigerated for prolonged periods.

If you live alone and cook for yourself, be extra careful – always check and abide by cooking times and use-by dates.

GOOD FOOD GUIDE

Be especially careful with meals if you can't taste or smell as well as you used to. These tips will help you to stay safe and well.

- Don't 'cook by taste' – always follow recommended cooking times and temperatures.
- Invest in a meat thermometer to test temperature on the inside of large joints or, especially, poultry.

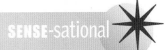

- Make sure that ready meals and any foods that are being re-heated are properly cooked through and piping hot.
- Maintain scrupulous kitchen hygiene; always wash your hands before preparing food.
- Keep raw meat and fish covered, on the bottom shelf of the fridge, and well away from any vegetables or cooked foods.
- Refrigerate any prepared items that you are not going to eat immediately
- Set your fridge and freezer to the recommended temperatures, and buy a fridge thermometer to ensure all perishable food is stored at 5°C (41°F) or below.
- Defrost frozen food thoroughly before cooking it.

BEWARE OF BLAND

A condition dubbed 'ageing anorexia', in which people progressively lose weight as they age, has been linked to a reduced sense of smell. It can get worse when people enter retirement homes, says Johan Lundstrom of Chicago University's Institute for Mind and Biology. He blames the often flavourless meals. If residents with a reduced sense of smell eat foods that 'taste like porridge,' he says, 'the only sensory information they receive about what they are eating is texture and basic taste, but no flavour.' As a result, they eat less and less. It's a malaise that may be more widespread. In the UK, where institutional food is notoriously bland, up to 60 per cent of elderly patients in NHS hospitals are malnourished, according to recent reports.

SMELLING DANGER

In the home, fire and gas are other potential hazards. Most people wake up if fire breaks out at night, as smell is the only sense that doesn't sleep, so those who can't smell are especially vulnerable. Fit a good smoke alarm on every floor and keep a fire blanket next to the cooker.

What about gas? Natural gas is odourless, but because gas leaks are so dangerous, risking both poisoning and explosions, gas companies deliberately add a strong, unpleasant smell so that it can be detected early. If you can't smell and you have the option, choose an electric oven and hob rather than a gas one, and oil-fired or electric heating. If not, fit a good quality natural gas detector that gives an early warning of a leak. Some can be linked to the gas supply to automatically cut it off – which is especially helpful if a leak occurs while you're out, so you don't walk into a house full of gas while unaware of the danger. Detectors are available from specialist security or electrical retailers; prices for basic models start at around £13. You can also get detectors for propane, butane and LPG if you use gas cylinders, for example, on a boat.

CHEMICAL ALERT!

If you don't have a good sense of smell, be careful when using household cleaners (especially bleach), garden chemicals, or paints in areas that are not well-ventilated. In particular, avoid paints that are high in VOCs (volatile organic compounds); they are often toxic and can make you feel giddy or nauseous if you're unaware of the odour and stay too close to them for too long. Make sure you read the warning labels on such products. If you're exposed to chemicals at work – and your loss of smell means that you could not detect a potential problem – contact your company's health and safety officers to discuss how to minimise the risks.

pinpoint the cause

While taste and smell can become blunted as we get older, any loss tends to be partial and there are many ways to compensate and perhaps even prevent or reverse the decline. So, pay your GP a visit before you accept that losing these senses is an inevitable part of ageing.

Coughs and colds We all know that colds, flu and other respiratory infections may temporarily affect our senses of smell and taste. And sometimes smell receptors in the nose are damaged and sense loss persists, possibly because viruses interfere with receptor cell replacement. About 20 per cent of smell and taste disorders are due to viral infections, and are most likely to occur in middle age, with women affected more often than men. Most people have only a partial loss of smell, which may be accompanied by smell distortions – familiar things don't smell quite right – and sometimes they'll experience a constant foul taste or smell. After several months, smell loss may improve spontaneously.

Ear infections People who suffer from chronic infections and inflammation of the middle ear may also experience a blunting of their sense of taste, as was noted in a

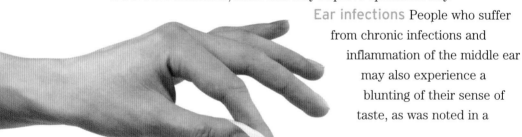

About 20 per cent of smell and taste disorders are due to viral infections, and persistent problems are most likely to occur in middle age, with women affected more often than men.

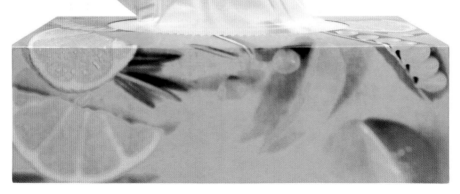

Japanese study, published in the US journal *Otology & Neurotology* in January 2007. As both hearing and taste could be affected, it is well worth ensuring that you get appropriate treatment for any ear infections.

Hayfever and other allergies There are several forms of rhinitis, a medical term which simply means that the membranes lining the nose are irritated and inflamed. Smell receptors are either blocked off or insensitive. It is most often due to allergies, such as hay fever, causing cold-like symptoms of a blocked, runny nose, sneezing and itchy eyes. Other causes include infections or pollutants and irritants such as cigarette smoke. There are numerous treatments that may alleviate some or all symptoms, so go and see your GP or, if the problem is severe, ask for a referral to an allergy specialist.

> There are many ways to compensate and perhaps prevent or reverse the decline, so pay your GP a visit before you accept that losing these senses is an inevitable part of ageing.

Sinusitis Inflammation of the mucosal lining of the sinus cavities – small air-filled spaces within the bones surrounding the nose – is usually due to infection, such as a cold, and generally clears up within a few weeks. But sometimes sinusitus, following an acute infection, can last for three months or more, especially if the person also smokes or has allergic rhinitis, nasal polyps, asthma or impaired immunity (as a result of AIDS, for example, or during chemotherapy). It may also occur with infection spreading from an infected tooth. The mucous lining of the sinus can become damaged, mucus builds up and drainage channels may be blocked. Loss of smell sensation often results, but as outlined in the next chapter, various treatments including medication and surgery, can be effective.

Polyps Nasal polyps are growths within the nasal passages that can cause loss of smell by blocking the nasal air passage, so that odour molecules in the air cannot reach the smell receptors at the top of the nose. Sometimes loss of smell is the first clue to polyps; as they are readily treatable, it's worth asking your doctor if this could be the problem. Unusually, this condition can cause loss of smell without any loss of taste, because retronasal olfaction is unaffected – smell molecules released when chewing can travel up the back route behind the nose, as the receptors themselves are unaffected.

Medications Many medicines, both prescription and over-the-counter, can interfere with the sense of smell. These include antibiotics, antihistamines, amphetamines, the contraceptive pill and the anti-impotence drug Viagra. Prolonged use of nasal decongestant sprays can also damage the nasal lining and lead to smell disorders, so read the instructions carefully and don't use beyond the prescribed number of days. If a prescription drug seems to be causing loss of smell or taste, talk to your GP to see if your prescription can be changed.

Neurological and psychiatric disorders Several nervous system disorders such as migraine, multiple sclerosis, Parkinson's or Alzheimer's disease are associated with smell and taste disorders, and are an often-overlooked cause of reduced appetite, weight loss and depression.

People suffering from psychiatric conditions such as schizophrenia, and anorexia may experience loss of taste and smell. Schizophrenia can also cause olfactory hallucinations – smelling something that isn't there, and this may also occur during epileptic seizures.

Head injury Across all age groups, the most common cause of complete loss of smell – anosmia – is head injury, most often sustained in road accidents. About one in twenty patients who have a head injury develop total anosmia, and another 30 per cent have reduced smelling capacity. They often also experience distorted smell – innocuous substances smell offensive – sometimes accompanied by unpleasant tastes.

The symptoms result from damage to the nerve fibres in the area at the top of the nose where smell receptors are located, or are sometimes due to direct injury to the brain. The more severe the head injury, the more likely it is that smell will be affected. Loss can sometimes be permanent or may take longer than a year to recover.

Surgery Some types of surgery can upset your sense of taste and smell, especially operations involving the ear, the nose or the sinuses, as well as radiotherapy for certain cancers of the head and neck. A tumour behind the nose or in the membranes surrounding the brain can also damage or even destroy your sense of smell.

SENSEalert !

SELF-PROTECTION

In some cases, lifestyle factors are responsible for loss of taste or smell, so the cure is within our control. Smoking is a common trigger as it irritates the nasal lining and can exacerbate symptoms of nasal polyps. Quitting will preserve these senses though it may take years to restore them fully. In addition, toxins such as insecticides and solvents can occasionally impair smell sense; although this is rare, it is worth being careful if handling either.

Other conditions Several medical problems that involve damage to the heart and blood vessels (cardiovascular system) are also linked with smell disorders, including heart attacks, stroke, diabetes and high blood pressure – indeed, some scientists think that smell disorders could be used to predict risk for these conditions.

Smell disorders can also occur with both malnutrition and obesity, vitamin A deficiency, hormonal disturbances and poor oral hygiene.

You may have tested your sense of smell or taste yourself, and perhaps identified some underlying risk factors that could compromise them.

your smart sense plan

This section has explained how you can best Protect and even enhance your smell and taste senses. You've learned how you can Assess them, and about the disorders that may affect them. You may have tested your sense of smell or taste yourself, and perhaps identified some underlying risk factors that could compromise them..

And you know that most problems do have an underlying cause, and that treatments are available to Correct certain conditions, prevent any further loss and perhaps improve your smell and taste capacity.

Your PACE strategy is taking shape. The next chapter describes the specialist tests that GPs and other medical experts use to diagnose various smell and taste disorders and outlines surgical solutions and other treatments.

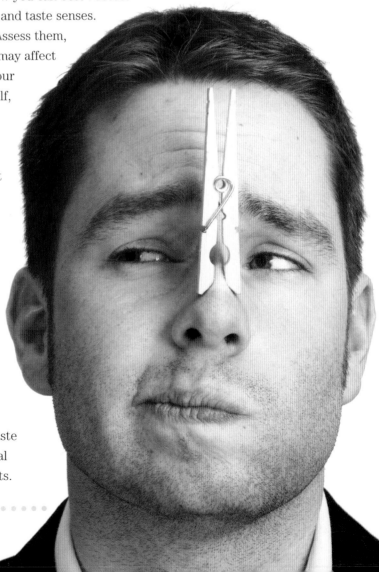

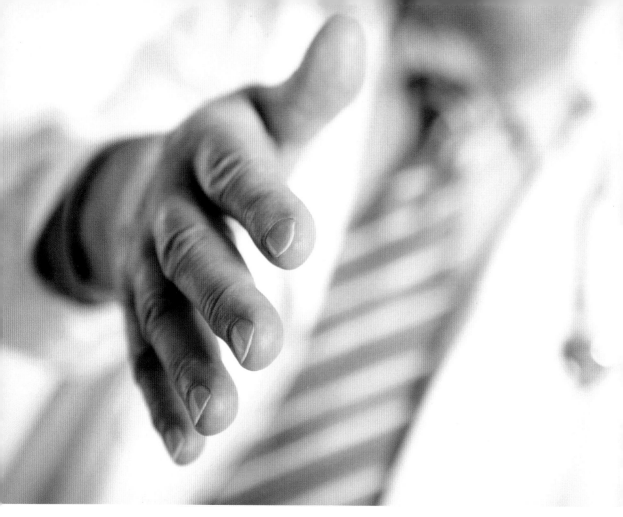

15   Smelling solutions

Sometimes, despite doing all you can to safeguard your senses, you will need medical advice. This chapter outlines how your GP and ENT specialists can treat loss of smell and taste.

Unless the loss of sensation is accompanied by some other obvious disorder, your doctor will probably start by asking you a few basic questions:

- Have you had a recent cold or upper respiratory infection?
- Do you smoke?
- Are you prone to sinus problems or allergies such as hay fever?
- Does the problem affect smell, taste or both?
- What medicines are you taking?

- When did you notice the first loss of sensation?
- Is it getting worse?
- Have you had any other associated symptoms?

Depending on your answers and any suspected cause, physical examination may include examining your nose, mouth and throat, looking for problems such as polyps or rhinitis. You may have your blood pressure taken or your urine tested (to check for diabetes), or a blood test.

Your doctor may be able to offer advice or treatment straightaway. If not, he or she may recommend further investigations such as X-rays, scans or specialised smell and taste tests, or may decide to refer you to an appropriate specialist, such as a neurologist or ENT (ear, nose, and throat) specialist for further assessment.

specialised tests

Occasionally an ENT specialist will suggest that a biopsy is taken to look at a tiny sample of your olfactory epithelium (the area at the top of your nose containing smell receptors). Otherwise, the diagnosis of smell and taste disorders relies on a series of specialised tests to measure the quality of your sensations.

Specialised tests are particularly useful for diagnosing taste and smell disorders because, unlike hearing or sight problems, most people have great difficulty assessing their senses of taste and smell and there is almost no correlation between how people describe their sense of smell and their actual performance in tests. One study of elderly people reported that 77 per cent of those with serious loss of smell described their sensation as 'normal'. In another study, 13 older people who claimed to have a normal sense of smell were found in tests to have none. That's not something that generally happens with, say, blindness.

SMELL TESTS

Your doctor may initially use a basic smell test (see page 210) where you see how close to your nose a distinctive smelling substance has to be before you detect it. Or he or she may test each nostril separately with a series of bottles containing common, readily-recognised smells such as lemon or coffee.

To check your ability to distinguish between a variety of different odours, you may be asked to take a 'scratch and sniff' test, sometimes called an UPSIT (because its formal name is the University of Pennsylvania

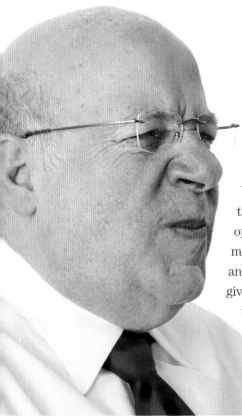

Smell Identification Test). This simple test takes about 10 or 15 minutes to complete, and can be done in the surgery or at home. It involves booklets containing a series of 40 scratch panels embedded with specific odours at the bottom right hand corner of each page. You simply scratch each panel with the tip of a pencil, then choose which smell it is most like, from four options given on the page, for example, does it smell most like (a) petrol (b) pizza (c) peanuts (d) rose. Your answers are then compared with standard responses given by people of the same gender and age band. This is the test that has been most commonly used for smell disorders; there is a similar mini-version known as the Pocket Smell Test. Since it was developed in the USA, it incorporates some smells that are not particularly familiar in Britain, such as pumpkin pie and root beer. A newer

You may be asked to take a 'scratch and sniff' test. This simple test takes about 10 or 15 minutes to complete, and can be done in the surgery or at home.

version that replaces these with 'British' smells was released in 2007, and a cross-cultural Brief Smell Test has been available in the UK for some time.

A more recent variant on the 'scratch and sniff' test are 'Sniffin' Sticks'. These look like ordinary felt-tip pens, but they are filled with fluids containing different odours. Sometimes the odours are presented on little discs – but the principle is the same.

THRESHOLD SENSITIVITY

Specialists might also suggest another test – called the Connecticut Chemosensory Clinical Research Center or CCCRC test – to check what is called your 'olfactory threshold' by finding out how well your nose can distinguish between water and the chemical butanol. For the test you will be presented with a pair of bottles, containing either water or the chemical, and asked to sniff each and try to identify the liquid in it.

The test is repeated using increasing concentrations of butanol until you can correctly distinguish the chemical from the water four times in a row. Each nostril is tested separately. The CCCRC test also has a second part in which you are asked to identify the specific smell in eight different bottles, from a list of common household and food items – anything from soap to cinnamon.

TASTE TESTS

Your specialist may use one of two fairly simple taste tests to rule out taste disorders, which are rare if you're not also suffering from loss of smell. The first is known as a 'taste and spit' test (or sometimes 'sip, spit and rinse'). As it suggests, you are asked to sample a series of liquids and identify basic tastes of salty, sweet, sour and bitter. Or you may be given taste strips, small pieces of filter paper soaked with specific flavours that are placed on the tongue. These also enable testing of different areas on the tongue.

effective treatment

No one has yet discovered a way to treat the gradual blunting of taste and smell that occurs in many people as they get older. (As explained earlier, this results from the slowing in the rate of replacement of taste and smell receptors that happens with age.) But, as you know, there are plenty of ways to give your senses a boost – for instance, by consciously exposing yourself to a variety of aromas or by treating your taste buds to a varied range of foods, as described in chapter 13. Doctors tend to take one of three basic approaches to smell and taste disorders:

- Changing your medicines Your GP can often prescribe an alternative if your medication interferes with taste or smell (see page 218).
- Treating the root cause Curing underlying medical problems, such as respiratory infections, can help to restore taste and smell.
- Nasal surgery An operation to remove obstructions is often effective. Loss of the senses of taste and smell is frequently temporary and the situation can improve with time. Olfactory cells are able to regenerate – though this may take months or even years (for example, following a head injury). In the meantime, try using stronger flavours and more herbs and spices in your cooking to compensate.

SENSEalert

WHEN FOOD TASTES TOO GOOD ...

Some smokers who stop enjoy renewed taste sensations so much that they put on more weight than they want to. This is easily remedied by keeping your diet healthy possible, and is no reason for weakening. Anecdotally, smoking may be linked to slimness, but a 2005 study of nearly 22,000 British people in *Obesity* showed that smokers tend to have more tummy fat – the kind that raises your risk of stroke and heart disease.

simple solutions

If an underlying medical condition is causing the problem, the solution may be straightforward. For example, your doctor may be able to alleviate your stuffy nose with decongestants, treat an ear infection (which can affect taste), or prescribe anti-allergic medications. Antihistamine drugs may help to reduce swelling and discharge in the case of allergies, rhinitis and sinusitis, and your sense of smell may rapidly return.

Any associated conditions, such as depression, diabetes or high-blood pressure, should be addressed, and this may also alleviate smell disorders. If you smoke, you will be advised to stop, and this may improve smell and taste sensations, though again it can take some time to regain full sensitivity.

If you are allergic to pet dander, the best treatment – sadly – is to remove the pet, especially if it's a cat, the most common cause.

ALLERGIES AND IRRITANTS

If your doctor thinks that your loss of smell or taste could be due to exposure to irritants, such as fumes or chemicals, he or she may suggest ways to avoid dust, pet dander (scurf) or other allergy-provoking substances. For example, someone with a dust allergy may be advised to dust with a damp cloth and vacuum more often, and to replace carpets and curtains with hard floor coverings and blinds. You can discover more information and get fact sheets from websites such as www.allergyuk.org.

If you are allergic to pet dander, the best treatment – sadly – is to remove the pet, especially if it's a cat, the most common cause. Up to 15 per cent of all people, and 35 per cent of asthma sufferers, are allergic to cats. It can take months or years before all traces of allergy provoking substances (fur, spit and dandruff proteins) are eradicated. It doesn't even have to be your own pet – many people's symptoms begin when they move to a new house that has previously had cats in residence. If the cause of an allergy isn't clear, you may be referred for allergy testing.

INFECTIONS AND BLOCKAGES

Your GP may occasionally prescribe antibiotics for respiratory or sinus infections due to bacteria (they don't work for virus infections), and once the infection has cleared up your sense of smell will often return. For persistent nasal discharge, a doctor may suggest that you try steam inhalation, a vaporiser or humidifier, to keep secretions loose and prevent the drying up of delicate membranes, especially overnight. As mentioned on page 216, chronic middle ear infections can also affect your sense of taste, so it is important to see your GP and get appropriate treatment.

If your smell sense is reduced as a result of nasal polyps, you will probably be referred for surgical treatment – see Surgery, page 230. In the meantime, your GP may prescribe corticosteroid drugs to reduce swelling in the nasal membranes – these may also help in some cases of rhinitis. Sometimes steroid tablets are used, and these can produce a successful return of smell sense. You may also find that avoiding dairy products (which are mucus-forming) may help to reduce congestion and improve your smelling capacity.

MOUTH PROBLEMS

Your GP can also treat mouth infections, and may advise you to see a dentist if there is any evidence of gum disease or other dental problems. If you have symptoms of dry mouth he or she may be able to prescribe an effective treatment to boost saliva flow and alleviate taste disturbances.

cutting**EDGE**

COULD NEW DRUG HELP TO PREVENT SMELL LOSS?

Loss of smell sensation in disorders such as rhinitis or chronic sinus disease is linked with the dying-off of smell-receptor cells in the nose at an increased rate, say researchers at Northwestern University in Chicago. The olfactory epithelium can generate new cells, but not as fast as normal, so the reduction in overall numbers may be what causes reduced smell sensitivity. The antibiotic minocycline could help because, as well as having anti-infective properties, it also appears to inhibit cell death in a number of other conditions. When they tested minocycline in mice, the researchers showed that the drug reduced the rate at which olfactory receptors died off. There is no evidence that it will also promote a regeneration of new cells, but the researchers believe it has potential for treating anosmia. While it has not been tested for its effect on smell loss in humans, it is currently undergoing trials for managing other neurological disorders associated with cell death (apoptosis).

Continued on p230 ➤

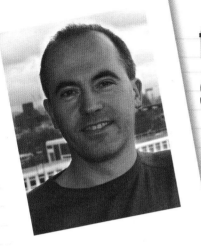

fighting back – in search of flavour

Mick O'Hare

Journalist Mick O'Hare loves good food and fine wines and is not the sort of man to relinquish his enjoyment of either without a fight. But a decade ago, he had no choice. The spicy curry he sat down to savour in front of the World Cup on television was utterly devoid of taste.

Mick had been suffering from a heavy cold, sore throat and blocked nose for the past week, so it wasn't surprising that his senses weren't as sharp as normal. Yet the loss he was experiencing felt different, he says. 'When you look in a fridge and it's empty, you can still see the fridge. This was like life without the fridge. There was an utter absence of anything, not even that unpleasant flavour of thick mucus.'

Curiosity compelled him to test his senses to the hilt in a bid to find anything, even foul smells, that might re-ignite the aromas and tastes he missed so much. 'I spent the next week sniffing everything from herb jars to dog muck – but nothing,' he says. 'It was terrifying.'

Mick now suspected something was seriously wrong and worried about the effect on the things in life he cherished. 'My wife and I were enthusiastic cooks and I was a member of CAMRA, the UK's real ale club. It was all suddenly meaningless.'

> 'I spent the next week sniffing everything from herb jars to dog muck – but nothing,' he says. 'It was terrifying.'

Mick waited. His cold got better but his senses of taste and smell did not return. He visited his GP's surgery but the locum who saw him was not helpful, he says. 'To be fair to her, it was more down to a lack of research into the subject by the medical profession in general. The stated line was "There is no cure", and she was just repeating that. She was sympathetic but told me to go away and live with it.

'I insisted on an ENT referral. The consultant poked a scope up my nose to have a look and got me to sniff bottles of smells I couldn't detect. He gave me a spray which didn't work and told me to accept the condition, saying he saw two or three people like me every year.'

THE HUNT BEGINS

It was not an opinion that Mick was prepared to accept. He got to know the medical terms – ageusia, the loss of the taste sense, and anosmia, the loss of smell – and scoured the internet for information. He discovered how taste and smell work together to enhance our enjoyment of food. And his own experience emphasised the difference between taste and flavour; after a few months, he gradually became able to distinguish bitter tastes such as green pepper and the sweetness of chocolate. 'Yet, agonisingly,' he recalls, 'I could only detect these as basic tastes. Aroma and the full flavour of foods were entirely absent.'

The prognosis was not good. Medical consensus was that the cold virus could have caused irreparable damage to his smell receptors. His own research confirmed that most experts believe that when the damage is too great, there is no effective treatment.

A DAILY STRUGGLE

Meals were agonising – 'I knew what I was missing' – but also a boring necessity: 'They are unavoidable, because if you don't eat, you die'.

By now, there were occasional odd flashes of smell but the odours were distorted. 'Wine smelled and tasted like kerosene and other odours – as disparate as car exhaust or perfume – blended into one acrid smell. To make matters worse I began to develop a chlorine-like taste in my mouth as well,' he says.

What also upset Mick was his friends' inability to understand what he was going through. 'One of the first things a fellow sufferer told me was that – unlike any other disability you might mention – people will openly laugh in your face when you tell them.

'But it's not amusing, it's dreadful. I found myself on the floor of the toilets at work one day, just crying my eyes out with the mental pain of my situation. I was so totally overwhelmed by what had happened.'

THE SCENT OF HOPE

Crucially, Mick didn't give up. When, via a web forum, he met a fellow sufferer who was recovering from anosmia, he pressed him for more information and found out about the Taste and Smell Clinic in Washington, DC, run by Dr Robert Henkin, a cognitive neurologist.

Mick visited the clinic in May 1999, 11 months after the virus first struck – and, like his earlier specialists, Dr Henkin concluded that the viral infection had caused the loss of sensation and distorted smells he experienced. But, to Mick's delight, this was not the end.

For 20 years Dr Henkin had been researching why, when the nose's smelling surface – the olfactory epithelium – is damaged, some patients recover their sense of smell spontaneously and others don't. He became increasingly convinced that the answer was associated with a substance present in nasal mucus – a growth factor called cyclic adenosine monophosphate (cAMP). cAMP appeared to be key to the regeneration of the epithelium and the millions of olfactory receptor cells it contains. But a sufficiently serious virus could knock out the cells that produce cAMP. 'The worse the smell loss, the lower the mucus cAMP,' explains Mick.

A WILLING GUINEA PIG

Dr Henkin then discovered that an existing medicine – theophylline (sometimes used in asthma to open up the airways) – could boost levels of cAMP. He tested it on patients who already had low levels and had not responded to other treatments. When Mick visited the clinic, Dr Henkin had published only one small clinical trial in which three out of four patients had reported improvement. It was hardly conclusive but Mick felt confident enough to go ahead. 'Because I couldn't spend the rest of my life anosmic and wondering "what if?", there was simply no other option,' he says.

'Early one morning I smelt coffee at work. That was the start – the moment when I could say recovery began. From there on it was perfume, tar, traffic, baking bread ... it was slow but it had begun.'

Dr Henkin treated him with theophylline in pill form, initially at a low dose (200mg), which was gradually increased to 600mg a day. He stayed at the clinic for a week, then returned home and continued taking the pills. The clinic kept in touch to monitor his treatment and see how he was responding.

'At first progress was slow. But within four months, hints of smell began to return,' says Mick. 'Early one morning I smelt coffee at work. That was the start – the moment when I could say recovery began. From there on it was perfume, tar, traffic, baking bread ... it was slow but it had begun.'

After 18 months, Mick's taste and smell levels seemed almost normal and Dr Henkin gradually decreased the theophylline dose. Mick hasn't been back to the clinic for two years. He now takes 150mg of theophylline every other day – partly as a precaution. 'Some people lose their taste and smell after stopping. Others don't. I'll take the tablets until both I and Dr Henkin feel it's OK to stop. It seems to have worked and I haven't suffered any side effects.'

Mick knows he is incredibly lucky. Theophylline may not work for everyone and is still not accepted by the medical establishment, although an increasing number of medical experts agree that viral anosmia is probably linked to regeneration of the olfactory epithelium, as Dr Henkin maintains.

And what has this 'miracle' cure meant for Mick? 'Everything!' he says. 'My life is restored in colour again. I savour every mouthful, every nuance. In many ways it has made me appreciate life more than I ever did.'

in search of a cure

Dr Robert Henkin makes a bold claim about taste and smell disorders. While most doctors say that little can be done and loss of taste and smell may have to be tolerated, he maintains that 'most patients can be treated effectively' – though success does depend on what prompted the loss.

The private Taste and Smell Clinic that he set up in 1986 in Washington DC claims outright cures or measurable improvements in more than 75 per cent of its cases. Patients undergo a battery of tests. Some would be carried out by any ENT specialist investigating a patient who had lost his sense of taste or smell; others, on saliva and nasal mucus, are a result of Dr Henkin's own research over more than 30 years.

His research suggests that there are specific proteins in saliva that act as growth factors and are essential for enabling taste buds to develop and mature. Trace metals, such as copper and zinc are also thought to play a crucial role. If the growth factors are lost your taste buds degenerate. Nasal mucus, he says, contains similar growth factors needed to promote olfactory epithelial (smelling) cells. These growth factors, in turn, are influenced not only by copper and zinc but also by calcium and magnesium.

For this reason, the clinic views results of tests on saliva and nasal mucus as crucial pointers to the causes and best treatment of the problem. It's what led Dr Henkin to prescribe theophylline to Mick O'Hare; he felt it would boost his deficient cAMP levels (cAMP is the growth factor that Dr Henkin believes is key to the regeneration of the olfactory epithelium and its millions of receptor cells). The clinic also uses other drugs to enhance growth factor, gene or nerve function.

SOME SCEPTICISM

So is theophylline a treatment for everyone who has suffered loss of smell following a virus? Professor Tim Jacob, a specialist in olfaction at Cardiff University, urges caution. 'There are no controlled trials that show the effectiveness of theophylline,' he says. 'Dr Henkin has looked at the effect of theophylline in unblinded, uncontrolled trials. No definite causative conclusions can be drawn from such studies.'

In April 2008 Dr Henkin presented the first formal study of theophylline treatment for smell disorders to the 121st annual meeting of the American Physiological Society, an apparently positive demonstration of its efficacy, although the study has not been peer reviewed. Professor Jacob remains sceptical and also points out that, with viral anosmia, 'recovery occurs naturally and spontaneously in about a third of all cases'.

It's also worth remembering that not all patients with smell loss have identifiable biochemical abnormalities. It's a long way to Washington DC, and treatment is likely to be costly. But the clinic undoubtedly offers hope to anosmia patients who have been told there is none, and for someone like Mick O'Hare, it's infinitely better than a scentless life.

surgery

Your doctor may advise surgery to treat nasal polyps, sometimes after pre-treatment with steroid drops to shrink their bulk. Polyp removal is a very straightforward operation that can usually be done under local anaesthetic. Similarly, if medications have not helped in chronic sinusitis, a minor operation can be performed to drain the sinuses. Again this is usually an outpatient procedure performed under local anaesthetic. In both cases you may have a head scan first so that the surgeon can be sure of the extent of the problem and the layout of your bones. These small operations can be highly successful in reducing obstructions and improving smell capacity.

Surgery to straighten the nose and allow normal air flow may also help to alleviate smell deficiencies in someone whose nose is crooked or whose septum – the sheet of bone and cartilage tissue dividing the two nostrils – is deviated. The two procedures may be combined.

general treatments

If there is an obvious cause for your loss of smell or taste sense, your doctor will want to treat it – and often sensations return to normal when underlying problems are resolved. And some types of smell or taste loss produce only temporary disturbances that resolve by themselves even without treatment. But you may also be advised about other steps that may help to speed up the return of your senses after specific treatment.

Zinc supplements may be recommended to treat loss of smell or taste (see pages 206-207), although clinical trials do not support their efficacy for treating either condition. Occasionally your doctor may recommend vitamin A, either by mouth or injection; vitamin A deficiency can cause loss of sense of smell, and there is limited evidence from animal experiments that synthetic vitamin A derivatives (retinoids) may boost repopulation of smell receptors after olfactory injury. But don't self-medicate. This treatment helps relatively few people, deficiency is rare and also excess vitamin A can be toxic.

perk up tired taste buds

If you do have reduced smell or taste sense, it's a good idea to enhance the stimulation you get, especially from food. As well as preserving sensation, simply enlarging your sensory repertoire can also help to boost fading senses and encourage their return. Here are some expert tips:

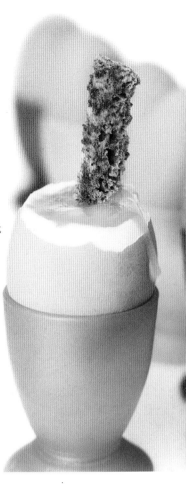

- Choose food ingredients or sauces with strong flavours (look at the umami-rich foods described on page 187).
- Don't neglect breakfast – your taste sensation is strongest in the morning.
- Experiment with new dishes – if you don't want to cook, try something you wouldn't normally have when eating out, or even a novel pre-prepared meal.
- Foods that look appealing usually taste better – aim for bright colours (which also tend to be healthier foods) and garnish dishes with herbs or a lemon or orange slice.
- Use more herbs and spices in cooking to add flavour.
- Use chilli and other spices to stimulate your chemical senses.
- Add stock or other flavourings to cooking water for rice and pasta, and to boost taste in casseroles and soups.
- Allow delicious cooking smells to circulate before a meal to stimulate your appetite.
- Serve foods warm – it makes them easier to taste.
- Chew food slowly to release more flavour.
- Don't drink scalding hot tea or coffee, which can damage your taste buds – give it a few minutes to cool down.

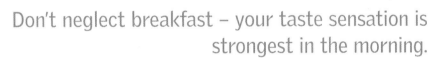

Don't neglect breakfast – your taste sensation is strongest in the morning.

- Sit up when you eat, it helps you to smell the food better.
- The setting in which you eat can make a difference – lay the table nicely and keep it free of clutter, use your best plates, maybe put a candle on the table or play some background music.

your smart sense plan

This chapter has outlined some of the ways you can Correct loss of taste or smell and revealed some novel ideas that offer hope that even age-related loss is not inevitable. And you are well aware of the enjoyment that results from keeping them in good working order. Unlike eyes and ears, which need a rest at times, the opposite is true for our senses of smell and taste, which tend to grow keener the more we consciously use them. So, feel free to surround yourself with gorgeous scents and delicious aromas and tempt your taste buds with a wide selection of delicious treats.

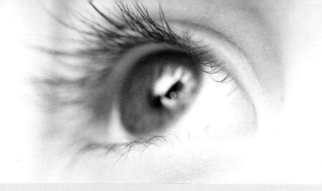
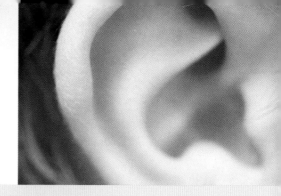

16 your smart taste & smell plan

There is much to suggest that your senses of taste and smell become sharper and more discerning the more you consciously use them. Which gives you every incentive to enjoy them to the full, sampling foods and wines, spoiling yourself with sensuous perfumes or simply revelling in the scents of summer.

It's also clear that there's often an underlying cause for fading sensations, that such causes may be both preventable and treatable, and that there's often something that your doctor can do to resolve the common problems.

Here's a quick summary to help you to ensure that all the PACE elements of your *Smart Sense Plan* for looking after and preserving your senses of taste and smell for life are in place.

Protect

- Are you fully aware of everyday tastes and smells? Can you remember the flavours in your last meal or snack? Can you describe what your nose has experienced in your home, in the garden or anywhere else today? 193
- Do you eat a wide range of foods, and experiment with new herbs and spices from time to time? 199
- Do you read packet labels to monitor your salt intake and take care how much you add during cooking or at the table? 198
- Do you present foods attractively and make mealtimes a pleasurable experience? 200
- Have you ever tried collecting smell memories? 200
- What are you doing to protect yourself against colds? 205
- Do you smoke? If so, are you trying to stop? 205
- Do you take good care of your teeth and oral hygiene? And do you visit a dentist regularly? 206
- Have you checked the list of 'enemies' and discussed with your GP how these might be affecting your senses of taste or smell? 180

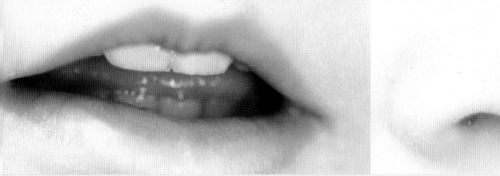

Assess
- What is your taster status? 197
- Are you aware of any loss of taste or smell? And have you taken our taste and smell tests? 209-210
- Have you any medical conditions, including dry mouth, that could increase your risk of smell or taste disorders? 211, 216-219
- Are you taking any medications that could affect taste or smell? 218
- Do you know what precautions you should take if your senses of taste or smell are impaired? 214-215

Correct
- If you have any smell or taste loss, have you had a proper diagnosis? 220
- Are you having treatment for hayfever, other allergies, or sinusitis? 216, 224
- If you suffer from diabetes or high-blood pressure – both linked to loss of smell and taste – are they under control? 224
- Are you aware of the links between loss of sensation and depression? 213
- Have you asked your doctor to review any medicines that might affect taste and smell? 218, 223
- What are you doing to boost your senses of taste and smell? 199, 230

Enjoy
- Can you remember the smells or tastes that delighted you as a child?
- How often do you now stop and savour the aromas and fragrances around you?
- How often do you eat and drink slowly enough to appreciate the rich bouquet of a good wine, subtle spices in an oriental dish or the scents and flavours of a sweet dessert?
- When did you last test fragrances – a perfume or aftershave – and buy something sensuous for yourself or a loved one?
- Can you remember the last time you enjoyed the delicious, evocative scent of newly mown grass?
- Are you continuing to guard against things that could damage your smell or taste sensitivity?
- What else could you do to improve your plan?

conclusions

By now, you will appreciate what a miracle of engineering our senses are, and how much they contribute to our safety, independence, well-being and enjoyment of life. You will understand how they function, what helps them to work optimally and what you need to do to maintain and preserve them.

You may have tailored your own *Smart Sense Plan* to your own specific needs and perhaps you're making changes in your life, monitoring your diet or activities to protect them more, taking the tests that will formally assess them and pinpoint any present or potential problems, taking note of expert advice or getting used to any treatment or aids that have been recommended. If so, you've achieved something that will bring life-long benefits.

What's more, the knowledge you have gained is something you will be able to use for ever. Our senses evolve and change throughout life, as the book explains. Most babies, for instance, are slightly longsighted, children's hearing is more acute than that of an adult, and their senses of taste and smell may be super-keen. The senses 'mature' when we grow up and, as we get older, they can change again.

So your *Smart Sense Plan* is not over when you've first devised it. A crucial part of the plan is to keep it going, so you are aware of any changes, which may occur so gradually that you barely notice them. That way you have the best chance of correcting them, if necessary, and keeping them in peak condition.

PRESERVING YOUR SENSES

One key message of this book is that loss of your precious senses as you get older is not inevitable. Indeed, there's plenty of evidence that the sensory losses that so many people accept as 'one of those things' may, in fact, be one of the so-called 'diseases of civilisation'.

This means that, like heart disease and cancer, these disorders may be becoming more prevalent because certain aspects of modern life are not conducive to good health. Human bodies evolved in an age when food was scarce and hunted, and physical fitness was a prerequisite for survival.

Like the rest of our bodies, our senses thrive on a natural lifestyle: enough exercise to keep us fit, a diet that includes lean, healthy protein, fresh fruits and vegetables, and fewer processed, fat, sugar and salt-laden foods that contribute calories but few worthwhile nutrients. You may have noticed that, in all three sections, the nutritional advice is very similar.

There are other aspects of 21st century life that are potentially harmful, such as noise, electronic screens and artificial light; research suggests that eyes benefit from the rest that pure darkness brings, and our aural senses which evolved when sound was less pervasive need periods of quietness to function well.

IN PERFECT HARMONY

We experience the world through all our senses, but we don't use them equally. Many eyesight and hearing problems stem from overload and over-stimulation. Many of us live in a visually-dominant, over-noisy world and it takes its toll.

It's a fact that today's generation of young people are likely to have poorer vision and hearing than their parents. They are also touch-deprived and may lose their senses of smell and taste earlier, because these senses are, by comparison, so under-used.

So we need to consider our senses in harmony, and to balance our sense system as a whole. For most of us, that means giving our eyes a rest from close work and computer screens, and our ears from damagingly high noise levels, and allowing our senses of taste, touch and smell to receive the stimulation for which they were designed.

It's time to take a break and go for a walk in the country, listen to the birds instead of the traffic, seek out fragrances that delight you and taste – really savour – your favourite food or wine. Because the ultimate message is that our senses are there to be enjoyed.

Following your *Smart Sense Plan* won't just keep your senses sharp, your vision vibrant, your hearing honed and your days full of fragrance and flavour, it will give you a better chance of living a long and healthy life. And a happy one.

glossary

[*Italicised* words have their own definitions]

accommodation The process by which the lens of the eye changes shape to enable focusing of images from varying distances.

acoustic neuroma A benign tumour of the *auditory nerve*.

age-related macular degeneration (AMD) An eye condition in which cells of the macula deteriorate, impairing vision.

anosmia Loss of the sense of smell.

antioxidant A nutrient that helps to counteract the damaging effects of *free radicals* within the body. Examples are vitamins A, C and E.

aqueous humour Fluid in the anterior chamber of the eye.

astigmatism A sight problem in which an irregularly-shaped *cornea* leads to multiple *focal points* and blurred vision.

atherosclerosis A disease in which arterial walls become thickened and hardened due to the build up of *cholesterol* and other deposits.

audiology The study of hearing and especially the diagnosis and treatment of hearing loss and rehabilitation for those affected.

auditory nerve The nerve conveying signals from the ear to the brain.

auroscope An instrument used to examine the outer ear.

blepharitis Inflammation of the eyelids.

carbohydrates Sugars and starches obtained from foods.

cataract Clouding of the lens of the eye, impairing sight.

cholesteatoma A cystic infection of the middle ear.

cholesterol Type of fat formed in the body from *saturated fat* in food and linked with heart disease and *atherosclerosis*.

choroid A dark pigmented layer lining the back of the eyeball.

ciliary muscles Tiny muscles that control the curvature of the lens of the eye, enabling it to focus incoming light rays onto the retina in the process of *accommodation*.

cochlea The spiral-shaped structure in the inner ear that contains hair cells responsible for sensing sound waves.

conductive hearing loss Hearing loss due to conditions in the outer or middle ear that interfere with sound wave transmission.

cones Type of light-sensitive *photoreceptor* in the *retina* responsible for colour and detailed daylight vision.

conjunctiva Transparent membrane covering the white of the eye and lining the upper and lower lids.

conjunctivitis Inflammation of the *conjunctiva* of the eye due to infection, allergy or irritants.

cornea The transparent protective covering of the front of the eye.

Decibel (dB) Unit of measurement of sound intensity.

diabetes A condition in which the body cannot regulate the levels of sugar in the blood.

eardrum The thin sheet of fleshy tissue that divides the outer from the middle ear cavities and transmits sound waves from outside to the *ossicles*. Known medically as the *tympanic membrane*.

Eustachian tube Tiny tube connecting the middle ear with the back of the nose and throat, to equalise pressure and drain secretions.

floaters Spots, blobs or strands that float about in the field of vision, due to shadows from debris in the *vitreous humour*.

focal point The point where light rays converge in the eye to create a clear image.

fovea The area in the middle of the *macula* of the retina that is most sensitive and responsible for detailed and colour vision.

free radicals Highly reactive chemical products formed during metabolism that may damage body cells and contribute to ageing and disease.

frequency A measure of the number of sound vibrations per second, which varies with the pitch.

glaucoma An eye disorder in which the optic nerve is progressively damaged, usually due to increased *intra-ocular pressure*. Without treatment glaucoma may lead to permanent vision loss.

glycaemic index (GI) A measure of how rapidly carbohydrates in food are converted to sugar in the body.

hyperacusis Hyper-sensitivity to certain noises.

hyperopia (hypermetropia) Long-sightedness. Close objects appear out of focus while distant images can be seen normally.

insulin The hormone produced by the pancreas that enables the body to metabolise glucose, and so controls blood sugar levels.

intra-ocular pressure The pressure of the fluid contained within the eyeball. A prolonged rise in pressure may lead to *glaucoma*.

iris The coloured circle surrounding the pupil of the eye.

lacrimal glands Tiny glands under the eyelid that produce tear fluid.

limbic system The area in the brain dealing with emotions and where smell impulses are received from the *olfactory receptors* in the nose.

lutein Natural pigment found in plants and also in the *macula* of the eye.

lysozyme A natural antibacterial substance that helps to counteract infection.

macula The area in the centre of the *retina* where light rays are focused, responsible for detailed vision.

melanin A type of pigment found in various cells in the body and responsible for the colour of skin, eyes and hair.

Ménière's disease A condition causing hearing loss and *vertigo*, due to a fluid build-up in the inner ear.

myopia Short or near-sightedness. Distant images appear blurred while close ones can be seen normally.

naso-lacrimal duct (tear duct) The tiny channel draining tears from the eye into the nose.

olfaction The medical term for the process of smelling. Orthonasal olfaction is the sensation from sniffing through the nose. Retronasal olfaction is the sense of flavour from smell molecules passing up the back of the throat into the nose when eating.

olfactory receptors Cells in the roof of the nose responsible for detecting smell.

omega-3 fatty acid An essential fatty acid found in oily fish, green leafy vegetables and some vegetable oils and generally insufficient in Western diets.

omega-6 fatty acid An essential fatty acid found in many vegetable oils and generally taken in excess in Western diets.

ophthalmoscope An instrument used to examine the eye.

optic nerve The nerve passing from the back of the eye to the brain, carrying signals from the *retina*.

ossicles Three tiny bones in the middle ear that transmit and amplify sound wave vibrations between the *eardrum* and the *cochlea*.

otosclerosis A cause of hearing loss, due to hardening of one or more of the *ossicles* in the middle ear, preventing transmission of soundwaves.

ototoxicity Damage to the ear from medicines or toxins.

photoreceptors Light-sensitive cells in the *retina*, either *rods* or *cones*.

presbyacusis Loss of hearing with age (spelt presbycusis in the USA).

presbyopia Difficult focusing close up, due to ageing.

proprioception The ability to sense the position of the body and the location of body parts.

pupil The dark part in the very middle of the front of the eye.

recruitment A symptom of hearing loss in which certain sounds are suddenly experienced at high intensity.

refraction Bending of light rays, necessary in the eye to produce a focal point for images of outside objects.

retina The layer of light-sensitive cells at the back of the eyeball.

retinopathy Disease of the small blood vessels in the *retina* of the eye, often due to *diabetes* (diabetic retinopathy).

rhinitis Inflammation of the mucous membranes lining the nose.

rhodopsin Light-reacting pigment contained in the rod cells of the *retina*.

rods Type of light-sensitive *photoreceptor* in the *retina* responsible for night vision.

saturated fat Type of fat found in foods of animal origin. High intakes increase blood *cholesterol* levels.

sclera The tough outer covering of the eyeball, seen as the white of the eye at the front.

semi-circular canals Three fluid-filled circular tubes in the *vestibular apparatus* of the inner ear responsible for detecting rotational movements.

sensorineural hearing loss Hearing impairment due to a problem with the conversion of soundwaves into electrical signals in the inner ear, or the transmission of nerve signals from the ear to the brain.

Snellen chart An eye chart with a series of rows of letters gradually reducing in size, used to test *visual acuity*.

tinnitus Ringing sensations or other unwanted noises in the ears unrelated to external sounds.

tonometry Tests to measure the pressure inside the eyeball.

trans fat Type of fat created during the processing of vegetable oils that acts like *saturated fat* in the body and is believed to be especially damaging to health.

tympanic membrane Medical term for the *eardrum*.

ultraviolet (UV) light Type of radiation found in sunlight but invisible to the human eye.

umami The fifth basic taste sensation, only recently recognised in the West.

vertigo A sensation of giddiness and spinning that results from disturbance to the *vestibular apparatus* in the inner ear or the balance centres of the brain.

vestibular apparatus The organs of balance in the inner ear, comprising *three semi-circular canals* and the *vestibule*.

vestibule The part of the inner ear that detects movement in a straight line and gravity. It has two parts, the saccule and the utricle.

visual acuity A measure of the sharpness of vision.

vitreous humour Jelly-like material in the posterior chamber of the eye.

yellow spot The *macula* of the eye.

zeaxanthin Natural pigment found in plants and also in the *macula* of the eye.

resources

Action for Tinnitus Research email: help@tinnitus-research.org tel: 020 7679 8907
www.tinnitus-research.org

Charity funding medical, scientific and social research into tinnitus and offering information
for patients and medical staff

AMD Alliance International Head Office: AMD Alliance International,
1929 Bayview Avenue, Toronto, Ontario, M4G 3E8, Canada email: info@amdalliance.org
Tel: +1-416-486-2500 extension 7505 www.amdalliance.org

Information on early detection, timely treatment, comprehensive rehabilitation and support
services for age-related macular degeneration

Association of Teachers of Lipreading to Adults (ATLA) Westwood Park,
London Road, Little Horkesley, Colchester, CO6 4BS email: ATLA@lipreading.org.uk
www.lipreading.org.uk

The professional association for teachers of lip-reading to adults who have become deaf, or
hard of hearing. Offers help to find local lip-reading classes

Blind Business Association Charitable Trust (BBACT) 29 Quantock Rise, Shepshed,
Leicestershire, LE12 9JR email: info@bbact.org.uk Tel: 0845 0450696 www.bbact.org.uk

Promotes self-employment for visually impaired people, including grants for people starting
their own business, to help with the purchase of essential equipment, and for education and
training

Blind in Business 4th Floor, 1 London Wall Buildings, London, EC2M 5PG
Tel: 0207 588 1885 www.blindinbusiness.org.uk

Charity offering help to blind and partially sighted people through employment and training
services

British Acoustic Neuroma Association (BANA) Oak House, Ransom Wood Business
Park, Southwell Road West, Mansfield, Nottinghamshire, NG21 0HJ tel: 01623 632 143
www.bana-uk.com

Information and support for people with acoustic neuroma

British Contact Lens Association Walmar House, 288/292 Regent Street, London,
W1B 3AL email: vfreeman@bcla.org.uk Tel: 020 7580 6661 www.bcla.org.uk

A charity representing eye care professionals and researchers. Offers information to the
public and help in finding a contact lens practitioner

British Tinnitus Association Ground Floor, Unit 5 Acorn Business Park,
Woodseats Close, Sheffield, S8 0TB email: info@tinnitus.org.uk Helpline 0800 018 0527
(Free, 9am – 5pm weekdays, answer phone at other times) www.tinnitus.org.uk

An independent charity offering information on tinnitus and related subjects for lay and
professional people. It also supports research and self-help groups

Driver and Vehicle Licensing Agency (DVLA) Drivers' Customer Services (DCS)
Correspondence Team, DVLA, Swansea, SA6 7JL email: drivers@dvla.gtnet.gov.uk
Tel: 0870 240 0009 www.dvla.gov.uk

For driver and vehicle enquiries including medical queries

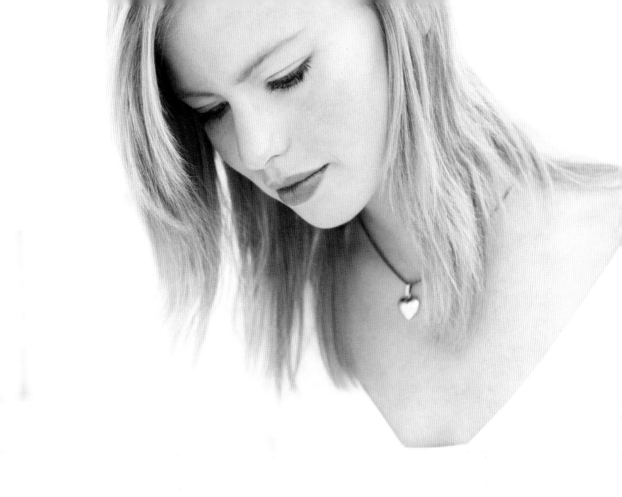

This book provides all the information you need to take action early, avoid unforeseen consequences and keep your senses in good working order.

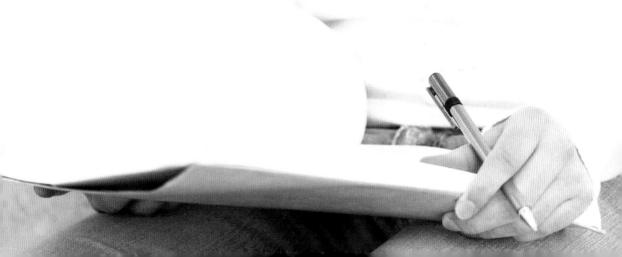

Healthcare Commission Helpline, Freepost, LON15399, London, EC1B 1QW
email: feedback@healthcarecommission.org.uk Helpline 0845 601 3012
ww.healthcarecommission.org.uk

Regulates and inspects private healthcare facilities including laser eye clinics

Hearing Concern 95 Gray's Inn Road, London, WC1X 8TX
email: info@hearingconcern.org.uk Tel: 020 7440 9871 HelpDesk: 0845 0744600
www.hearingconcern.org.uk

A national charity providing support, advice and information to deaf and hard of hearing
people

Hearing Dogs for Deaf People The Grange, Wycombe Road, Saunderton,
Princes Risborough, Buckinghamshire, HP27 9NS email: info@hearingdogs.org.uk
Tel: 01844 348 100 (voice & minicom) www.hearingdogs.org.uk

Provides hearing dogs to alert their deaf owners to sounds

Hyperacusis Network Post Office Box 8007, Green Bay, Wisconsin 54308, USA
email: earhelp@yahoo.com www.hyperacusis.net

US-based organisation offering information and support on hyperacusis and associated
symptoms to sufferers worldwide

Institute of Advanced Motorists IAM House, 510 Chiswick High Road, London, W4 5RG
Tel: 0208 996 9600 www.iam.org.uk

Road safety organisation offering DriveCheck Assessments and preparation for the Advanced
Driving Test

International Glaucoma Association 15 Highpoint Business Village, Henwood, Ashford,
Kent, TN24 8DH email: info@iga.org.uk Tel: 01233 648 170 (with SightLine)
www.glaucoma-association.com

An independent charitable organisation based in England offering patient information about
glaucoma in various languages

Learndirect Dearing House, 1 Young Street, Sheffield, S1 4UP
Tel: 0800 100 900 8am – 10pm Typetalk 18001 0800 100 900 Minicom 08000 568 865
www.learndirect.co.uk

Adult educational support including lip-reading courses

Macular Disease Society PO Box 1870, Andover, SP10 9AD
email: info@maculardisease.org Tel: 01264 350 551 Helpline 0845 241 2041
www.maculardisease.org

A self-help society providing information and practical support, with a nationwide network of
local support groups

Ménière's Society The Rookery, Surrey Hills Business Park, Wotton, Dorking, Surrey,
RH5 6QT email: info@menieres.org.uk Helpline 0845 120 2975 Minicom 01306 876 8057
www.menieres.org.uk

Charity offering support and information to members with Ménière's Disease

National Independent Bowel Cancer Screening Programme
Point Of Care Testing Ltd, Unit 5, Arbroath Business Centre, Dens Road, Arbroath, Angus,
DD11 1RS info@pocl.co.uk Tel 0845 603 5709 www.pocl.co.uk

Private testing for bowel cancer (carried out by post)

NHS Smoke free Free helpline 0800 0224332 – open 7 days a week, 7am to 11pm
www.gosmokefree.nhs.uk

Free help, resources, nicotine replacement products, local support groups and more

Royal College of Ophthalmologists 17 Cornwall Terrace, London, NW1 4QW
president@rcophth.ac.uk Tel 020 7935 0702 www.rcophth.ac.uk Downloadable guide to
laser surgery www.rcophth.ac.uk/about/public/laser

Professional body for eye specialists in the UK

Royal National Institute for Deaf People (RNID) 19-23 Featherstone Street, London,
EC1Y 8SL email: informationline@rnid.org.uk Tel: 020 7296 8000
Textphone 020 7296 8001 Information line (free) 0808 808 0123 Telephone hearing test
0845 600 5555 www.rnid.org.uk

The UK's largest charity for deaf and hard of hearing people

Royal National Institute of Blind People (RNIB) 105 Judd Street, London, WC1H 9NE
email: helpline@rnib.org.uk Tel: 020 7388 2525 Helpline 0845 766 9999 www.rnib.org.uk

Help and support for blind and visually impaired people

UK Synæsthesia Association PO Box 6258, Leighton Buzzard, LU7 0WP
email: uksynaesthesia@hotmail.com Tel: 01253 798330 www.brighton-breezy.co.uk

A non-profit making organisation run by and for people with an interest in synæsthesia –
when people experience a sense with a different sense, such as a sound invoking a colour.

Vestibular Disorders Association PO Box 13305, Portland OR 97213-0305, USA
Tel: +1-503- 229-7705 www.vestibular.org

US-based organisation that provides information, resources, support, and advocacy for people
with inner ear disorders

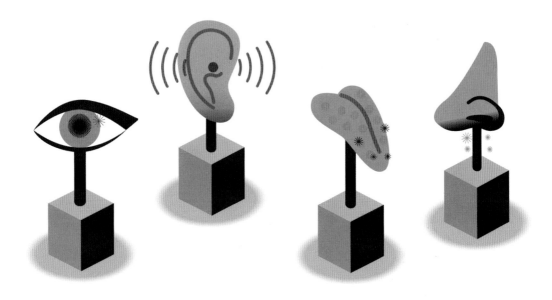

index

A

acamprosate 160

acoustic neuroma 149, 163

acoustic trauma 128

adenoids, enlarged 145, 162

adrenaline 28

Age-Related Eye Disease Study (AREDS) 41

age-related macular degeneration (AMD) 29, 31, 32, 38, 84, 92-97

  alcohol intake and 40

  diet and 42, 46, 93

  dry AMD 93-94

  effects 92

  environmental factors 93

  family history of 92, 93

  gender and 46

  genetic factors 93

  macular dystrophy 92, 93

  predictor of strokes and heart attacks 44, 46

  protection against 39, 40, 44, 45

  risk factors 46, 47

  smoking and 46, 47

  symptoms 93

  testing for 95-96

  treatment 94, 96-97

  wet AMD 94, 96

ageing

  and eye problems 19, 29, 38, 50, 65-66, 67, 102-107

  and hearing impairment 117, 120, 124, 133, 137, 148

  and taste/smell impairment 179-180, 188-189, 192, 199, 206, 208-209, 210, 212, 215, 216, 221

ageing anorexia 215

ageusia 210, 227

albinos 27

alcohol 189

  abuse 27

  adverse effects 40

  dehydration 212

  for eye health 39-40

  for hearing health 134

  super-tasters and 197

  wine tasting 193, 195

alcohol sniff test (AST) 210

allergies 30, 81, 145, 217, 224-225

alpha-lipoic acid 137, 207

Alzheimer's disease 91, 180, 218

amblyopia 65

amino acids 186-187

amphetamines 218

Amsler Grid 95-96

anecortave acetate 91

angiotensin-converting enzyme (ACE) inhibitors 211

anorexia 218

  ageing anorexia 215

anosmia 199, 212, 214, 218, 225, 226-228, 229

anti-VEGF therapy 94, 96

antibiotics 147, 158, 159, 218, 225

antidepressants 160, 211, 213

antihistamines 81, 211, 218, 224

antioxidants 38, 39, 40, 41, 94, 134, 135, 207

  supplements 45, 136-137, 207

apoptosis 225

appetite loss 213, 214, 218

artificial tears 80, 82, 83

aspirin 137, 146, 147

Assistive Listening Devices (ALDs) 166

astigmatism 66-67, 68-69

  contact lenses for 71

G

H

I

J,K,L

N

nasal discharge 225

nasal polyps 217, 221, 225, 230

nasal surgery 223, 230

near sight *see* shortsightedness

Neitz, Professor Jay 55

night driving 26-27, 30, 107

night vision 26-27, 39

noise

    harmful 118, 120, 128-130

    health-related problems 127

    limiting exposure to 118, 128-129, 131

    measurement 118, 119

    prolonged exposure to 127, 148

    secondhand noise 127-128

    in the workplace 127, 128

non-steroidal anti-inflammatory drugs
    (NSAIDs) 86, 147

noradrenaline 213

nuisance odour respirators 206

nutritional deficiencies 206

O

obesity 21, 197

    and eye problems 31, 44

    risk factor for AMD 46

    and smell disorders 219

odour

    molecules 183, 217

    recognition 185

    see also index entries beginning 'smell'

O'Hare, Mick 226-228, 229

olfaction 182-183

    orthonasal 182, 183

    retronasal 182, 183, 212, 217

olfactory bulb 185

olfactory cells 223, 225, 229

olfactory epithelium 184, 221, 225, 227

olfactory hallucinations 218

olfactory receptor neurones 184, 185

olfactory threshold 222

olfactory tract 185

omega-3 fatty acids 42, 46, 82

omega-6 fatty acids 42, 46

ophthalmic medical practitioners 52

ophthalmic surgeons *see* ophthalmologists

ophthalmologists 52, 75, 83-84

ophthalmoscopes 51, 53, 83, 90

    indirect ophthalmoscopy 83

    slit-lamp ophthalmoscopy 84

optic nerve 22, 29, 89

optic neuritis 110

opticians *see* dispensing opticians

optometrists 52

oral hygiene 189, 206, 211, 219

orthoptists 52

otitis media 145, 158, 162

otoacoustic emission test 156

otolaryngologists 154

otorhinolaryngologists 154

otosclerosis 148, 162-163

ototoxic medications 146-147, 158

P

Parkinson's disease 180, 218

pegaptanib 96

perfumery 202-203

perimetry 90

pet dander 224-225

phacoemulsification 86

phones, for the hard-of-hearing 157, 166

photodynamic therapy (PDT) 94

photorefractive keratectomy (PRK) 75, 77

pink eye *see* conjunctivitis

pink noise generators 160, 161

placebo fragrances 204

depth perception 103, 105

good lighting, ensuring 105, 108

hazards 104

home safety 104

multifocals, dangers of 105

stairs 103, 105

tuning fork tests 155-156

tunnel vision 89

tympanoplasty 162

U,V

ultraviolet (UV) light 38, 64, 73

umami 186, 199, 209

vaporisers 225

vascular endothelial growth factor (VEGF) 94

venous insufficiency 138

vertigo 127, 138, 147, 149, 150, 159, 161-162

benign paroxysmal positional vertigo (BPPV) 161-162

therapies for 161-162

Vertigoheel® 138

vestibular rehabilitation therapy (VRT) 162

Viagra 218

viral infections 158, 216, 227

vision

aids for partially sighted people 108-109

binocular 52

blurred 21, 30, 33, 34, 59, 60, 65, 80, 92, 93

colour vision 24, 54, 108

contrast sensitivity 103, 105

depth perception 103, 105

double 21, 52, 65, 79, 85

night vision 26-27, 39

peripheral 89, 90, 92, 106

see also sight

vision loss

at the periphery 24

long-distance 45

partial 21

sudden 21, 79

see also age-related macular degeneration (AMD); blindness; glaucoma

visual acuity (VA)

impaired 57, 79

normal 56

testing 53, 56-57

20/20 vision 56, 57

visual overload 193

vitamin A 40, 137, 219, 230

vitamin C 40, 41, 45, 136, 137

vitamin D 135

vitamin E 40, 41, 45, 137, 207

vitreous humour 23, 97

volatile organic compounds (VOCs) 215

W

watery eyes 21, 79, 80, 84

Wayfinder Access software 111

weight loss 218

white noise generators 160

workstation, eye-friendly 36-37

Y,Z

yellow spot see macula lutea

yoghurt 189

Yung, Matthew 173

zeaxanthin 38, 39

zinc 40, 41, 45, 136, 206-207, 229, 230

Keep Your Senses Sharp was originated by The Reader's Digest Association Limited, London

First edition copyright © 2008
The Reader's Digest Association Limited,
11 Westferry Circus, Canary Wharf, London E14 4HE

We are committed both to the quality of our products and the service we provide to our customers. We value your comments, so please do contact us on 08705 113366 or via our website at
www.readersdigest.co.uk

If you have any comments or suggestions about the content of our books, email us at
gbeditorial@readersdigest.co.uk

Colour origination Colour Systems Limited, London

Printed and bound in China

Reader's Digest Project Team

Editor Rachel Warren Chadd
Art editors Jane McKenna, Simon Webb
Assistant editors Helen Holmes, Henrietta Heald
Picture researcher Rosie Taylor
Proofreader Ron Pankhurst
Indexer Marie Lorimer

Reader's Digest General Books

Editorial director Julian Browne
Art director Anne-Marie Bulat
Managing editor Nina Hathway
Head of book development Sarah Bloxham
Picture resource manager Sarah Stewart-Richardson
Pre-press account manager Dean Russell
Product production manager Claudette Bramble
Senior production controller Katherine Bunn

Paperback codes
Concept code UK2490/IC
Book code 400-385 UP0000-1
ISBN 978 0 276 44389 3
Oracle code 250012452S.00.24